PREVENTING VIOLENCE

The Past, Present and Future of
the Public Health Approach

Keir Irwin-Rogers, Luke Billingham,
Alistair Fraser, Fern Gillon, Susan McVie
and Tim Newburn

First published in Great Britain in 2025 by

Policy Press, an imprint of
Bristol University Press
University of Bristol
1–9 Old Park Hill
Bristol
BS2 8BB
UK
t: +44 (0)117 374 6645
e: bup-info@bristol.ac.uk

Details of international sales and distribution partners are available at
policy.bristoluniversitypress.co.uk

© Keir Irwin-Rogers, Luke Billingham, Alistair Fraser,
Fern Gillon, Susan McVie, Tim Newburn 2025

The digital PDF and ePub versions of this title are available open access and distributed under the terms of the Creative Commons Attribution-NonCommercial-NoDerivatives 4.0 International licence (https://creativecommons.org/licenses/by-nc-nd/4.0/) which permits reproduction and distribution for non-commercial use without further permission provided the original work is attributed.

British Library Cataloguing in Publication Data
A catalogue record for this book is available from the British Library

ISBN 978-1-4473-7384-1 paperback
ISBN 978-1-4473-7385-8 ePub
ISBN 978-1-4473-7386-5 ePdf

The right of Keir Irwin-Rogers, Luke Billingham, Alistair Fraser, Fern Gillon, Susan McVie and Tim Newburn to be identified as authors of this work has been asserted by them in accordance with the Copyright, Designs and Patents Act 1988.

All rights reserved: no part of this publication may be reproduced, stored in a retrieval system, or transmitted in any form or by any means, electronic, mechanical, photocopying, recording, or otherwise without the prior permission of Bristol University Press.

Every reasonable effort has been made to obtain permission to reproduce copyrighted material. If, however, anyone knows of an oversight, please contact the publisher.

The statements and opinions contained within this publication are solely those of the authors and not of the University of Bristol or Bristol University Press. The University of Bristol and Bristol University Press disclaim responsibility for any injury to persons or property resulting from any material published in this publication.

Bristol University Press and Policy Press work to counter discrimination on grounds of gender, race, disability, age and sexuality.

Cover design: Lyn Davies Design
Front cover image: Getty/temizyurek

Contents

List of figures and tables	v
About the authors	vi
Acknowledgements	vii

Introduction	**1**
Scope	2
Trends in violence	5
The causes of interpersonal violence	8
The public health approach to violence prevention	14
Researching the public health approach to violence prevention	17
Structure and style	21

PART I A short history of the public health approach to violence prevention

1	**Roots and shoots of the public health approach to violence prevention**	**27**
	Early roots of the public health approach to violence prevention	28
	The origins and development of Scotland's public health approach	29
	The journey toward a public health approach: England and Wales	37
	Conclusion	42

2	**Recent developments in England and Wales**	**44**
	From a crescendo of calls to official orthodoxy	46
	Institutionalisation of the public health approach: VRUs, YEF, and the Serious Violence Duty	55
	What did the public health approach come to be?	63
	Conclusion	71

PART II	**Violence Reduction Units**	
3	**Bedding in, reaching out**	**75**
	Establishing the Violence Reduction Units	76
	Pressure to spend money in haste	79
	Building legitimacy and securing trust	81
	Multi-agency working	83
	The Serious Violence Duty	94
	Engaging with communities and young people	99
	Conclusion	102
4	**Aiming upstream, slipping downstream**	**104**
	Commissioning interventions to reduce violence	105
	Influencing government and institutional policies	123
	Conclusion	129
PART III	**Looking ahead**	
5	**Where should we go from here?**	**133**
	Preventing violence through coordinated action across the Four Is	134
	Recent violence prevention initiatives: applying a Four Is lens	138
	Advancing a truly holistic public health approach to violence prevention	141
	The future of Violence Reduction Units	146
	Limitations and potential pitfalls	151
	Conclusion	153

Appendix: Q-grid activity from VRU workshop	156
Notes	162
References	164
Index	190

List of figures and tables

Figures

1	Number of violent incidents: annual estimates, England and Wales, 1982–2024	5
2	Homicide incidents: England and Wales and Metropolitan Police Service, 1990–2023, indexed to 1990	6
3	Hospital admissions for assault with sharp objects, England and Wales, age group 0–24, 2012–13 to 2023	7
4	Violence in London, per 1,000 people, by type, 2002–19	8
5	An ecological framework for understanding the factors linked to violence	11
6	The Four Is framework	16
A.1	Group A Q-grid	157
A.2	Group B Q-grid	157
A.3	Group C Q-grid	158
A.4	Group D Q-grid	158
A.5	Group E Q-grid	159
A.6	Group F Q-grid	161

Tables

1	VRU director backgrounds and first-year funding	77

About the authors

Keir Irwin-Rogers is Senior Lecturer in Criminology at The Open University.

Luke Billingham is a youth and community worker at Hackney Quest and Research Associate at The Open University.

Alistair Fraser is Professor of Criminology at the University of Glasgow.

Fern Gillon is Research Assistant at the Scottish Centre for Crime & Justice Research at the University of Strathclyde.

Susan McVie is Professor of Quantitative Criminology at the University of Edinburgh.

Tim Newburn is Professor of Criminology and Social Policy at the London School of Economics.

Acknowledgements

We would like to express our thanks to all the organisations, and the 189 policy makers, senior leaders, frontline professionals and young people, who supported and participated in the project, 'Public Health, Youth and Violence Reduction' (PHYVR), funded by the Economic and Social Research Council (ESRC), between 2019 and 2023.

A special thank you to the directors of all 21 Violence Reduction Units in England, Wales and Scotland, who generously gave their time for interviews, online workshops, and our face-to-face conference in London in September 2023.

Thank you to the book's informal and formal peer reviewers for providing encouraging and constructive comments on the initial proposal and successive drafts.

Finally, we extend heartfelt thanks to our families and friends – this book would not have been possible without their patience, encouragement, and support throughout the period of research and writing.

Introduction

Violence is an enduring part of human history and one of the most harrowing aspects of humanity. While no society has ever managed to eradicate violence in all its forms, levels and types of violence have varied significantly across time and place. In the United Kingdom (UK) at the time of writing, the prevention of interpersonal violence is a central political priority. In May 2024, the Labour Party swept to power on the promise of a 'mission-driven government'. Tackling violence is one of its five core missions, with Labour pledging to 'take back our streets by halving serious violent crime' (Labour, 2024). This book is based on the premise that this type of mission can be achieved. There is nothing preventing us from better understanding why serious interpersonal violence occurs and converting this knowledge into action to bring about much safer societies.

The fundamental argument we make in this book is that we can move towards less violent societies by advancing a public health approach to violence prevention. Our main aim is to provide a novel and comprehensive framework for the public health approach, and to show why it offers a transformative path towards a low-violence society. When the term 'public health approach' has been used in recent years – by politicians, journalists, professionals, or academics – it often lacks sufficient explanation. It has become clear to us that people are using the term to mean very different things. Despite its potential, we argue that the way the approach has been commonly understood and implemented in England and Wales is severely limited. A large part of this book is therefore devoted to exploring these limitations and charting an alternative and more fruitful path ahead.

We also aim to provide an in-depth account of the development of Violence Reduction Units (VRUs) in England and Wales, which have become a key component of the public health approach. The long-term future of these units is uncertain, and we hope this book offers a timely insight into their work and potential value.

Broadly, we seek to address the following questions:

- What is the nature and scale of violence in England and Wales? What are the main causes of violence? (Introduction)
- What are the origins of the public health approach to violence prevention and how did it develop over time? What are the main strengths and limitations associated with the way the public health approach is currently conceptualised and implemented in England and Wales? (Part I: Chapters 1 and 2)
- What role do VRUs play in advancing the public health approach? What challenges and opportunities do these units face? (Part II: Chapters 3 and 4)
- How can a truly holistic public health approach to violence prevention be conceptualised? What steps are needed to turn this vision into reality in England and Wales? (Part III: Chapter 5)

In this introductory chapter we set the scene by examining the nature and scale of interpersonal violence in England and Wales. We look closely at London, as it is commonly the source of public and political concern around violent crime. Next, we review what current research suggests about the causes of violent crime, before introducing the central topic of this book: the public health approach to violence prevention. This section provides an initial insight into the development of the public health approach, which we pick up in much greater detail in Part I. We then outline the research on which this book is based: a three-year project involving a collaboration of academics across four universities in England and Scotland, funded by the Economic and Social Research Council (ESRC).[1] Lastly, we discuss the book's overall structure and style. We begin with some notes on the book's scope.

Scope

The parameters of our enquiry are set along two main lines: a focus on 'youth violence' and a geographic concentration on England. In this section, we explain why.

Introduction

'Youth violence'

The central topic of this book is the public health approach to violence prevention. As the public health approach has primarily focused on preventing violence by young men – particularly in England and Wales in recent years – this subtype of interpersonal violence features most squarely in our analysis. While this is commonly referred to as 'youth violence', for a number of reasons, we prefer the term 'violence affecting young people'.[2] In short, this is because the term 'youth violence' tends to both narrow and blur people's focus, while unhelpfully twinning 'youth' with the negative and stigmatising concept of 'violence' (see further Billingham and Irwin-Rogers, 2022, pp 5–12).

There are many other types of behaviour that fall within the umbrella term of 'violence', including, for example, intimate partner violence, family violence, sexual violence, and physical violence committed by and against adults. The reason this book focuses squarely on violence affecting young people is threefold:

- credible data (discussed later) indicate that this form of violence has risen in recent years (as has young people's fear of violence, see Youth Endowment Fund, 2024a);
- this issue has recently received serious attention from policy makers, and there is scope for building on current policy initiatives;
- the book is based on a research project that focused on violence involving young people, at both policy and community levels.

Although our intention is to better make sense of violence affecting young people and identify ways of preventing it, this necessarily entails a consideration of 'structural violence'. By this we mean the violence or harm generated by social structures, including institutions, systems, and policies. For example, the failure of successful UK governments to tackle soaring housing costs is one of the most obvious forms of structural violence that plunges millions of children into poverty each year (Child Poverty Action Group, 2024b).

Geographic focus

The vast majority of the research on which this book is based took place in England and Wales, as this is where the now 20 regional VRUs were established. However, Part I extends its scope beyond England and Wales to include Scotland and the United States (US). These countries have seen significant progress in the development of public health approaches to violence prevention, preceding the formal adoption of the public health approach in England and Wales. When we refer to statistics on violence (including in the following section), these relate sometimes to England and Wales, sometimes to the UK, and sometimes to England alone. This reflects the way in which these statistics are collated in national surveys, and by organisations such as police forces and the National Health Service (NHS).

Generalisability

While our primary intention is to advance public health approaches to the prevention of violence between young people, the essence and core components of the public health approach that we propose – for example, recognising that drivers of violence operate at distinct levels (societal, community, relational, and individual levels) and that action to reduce violence should take place at national and local levels – could equally be applied in efforts to prevent other types of violence (see further Bellis et al, 2017). We hope, therefore, that this book will prove useful to people working to prevent many different forms of harm and violence.

Similarly, while the main purpose of the book is to advance the public health approach to violence prevention specifically in England and Wales, we believe many of the arguments we make in this book are likely to apply more broadly. Judgements about the broader applicability of the findings and recommendations in this book, however, require a detailed knowledge and understanding of national and local factors that may affect generalisability, and are therefore best made by those living and working in other places.

Trends in violence

Levels and types of violence have varied considerably throughout history and across populations. Some scholars, including Pinker (2011, 2018), have argued that we are living through the most peaceful period in human history. Although there are occasional spikes in violence due to specific conflicts, taken as a whole and viewed across centuries and millennia, rates of violence have steadily declined over time (for a critique of Pinker's thesis, see Dwyer and Micale, 2021). In keeping with trends in many countries around the world, best estimates suggest the numbers of incidents of violent crime in England and Wales are currently at an all-time low (see Figure 1).

Looking only at the trend for all types of violence combined into a single category and over a prolonged period, however, masks variation for particular types of violence over shorter timeframes. While Figure 1 shows that the general trend for violence in England

Figure 1: Number of violent incidents: annual estimates, England and Wales, 1982–2024

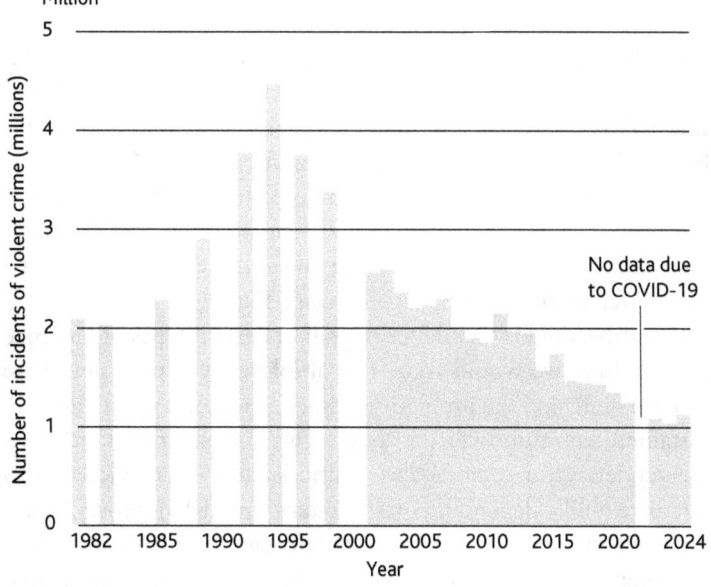

Source: Office for National Statistics (2024a)

Figure 2: Homicide incidents: England and Wales and Metropolitan Police Service, 1990–2023, indexed to 1990

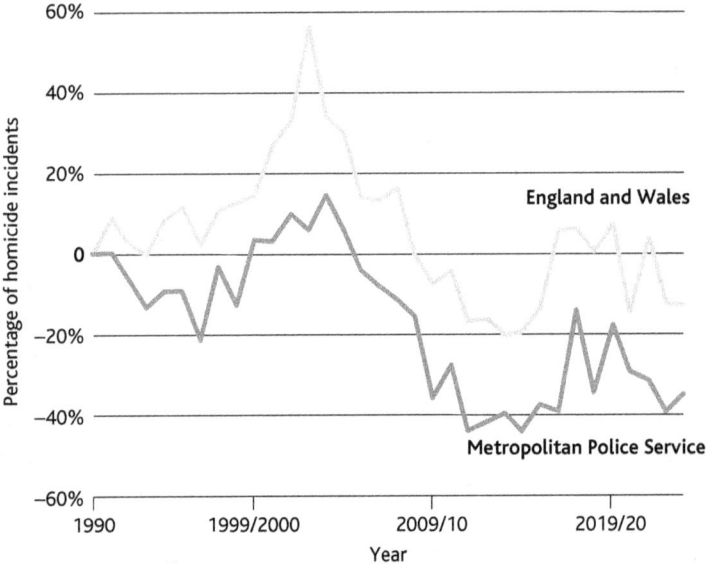

Source: Office for National Statistics (2024b)

and Wales is one of reduction, in recent years, some metrics for serious violence indicate that certain forms of serious violence underwent a significant increase during the years 2014–19, before declining again (see Figure 2 and Figure 3).

Examining data for London in particular – the city where concerns around interpersonal violence are often acute – shows that trends can vary in their nature and scale when broken down into different subtypes of violence (see Figure 4).

Regardless of how violence overall or certain types of violence are trending, we would argue that absolute levels of violence are still too high, and the problem of violence requires significant and sustained attention over the long term. This is important given the tendency for societal and political attention to violence to fluctuate wildly depending on short-term trends. Moreover, while objective measures of violence are important, people's perceptions of violence – and fear of violence in particular – are also notable from a quality-of-life perspective.

Figure 3: Hospital admissions for assault with sharp objects, England and Wales, age group 0–24, 2012–13 to 2023

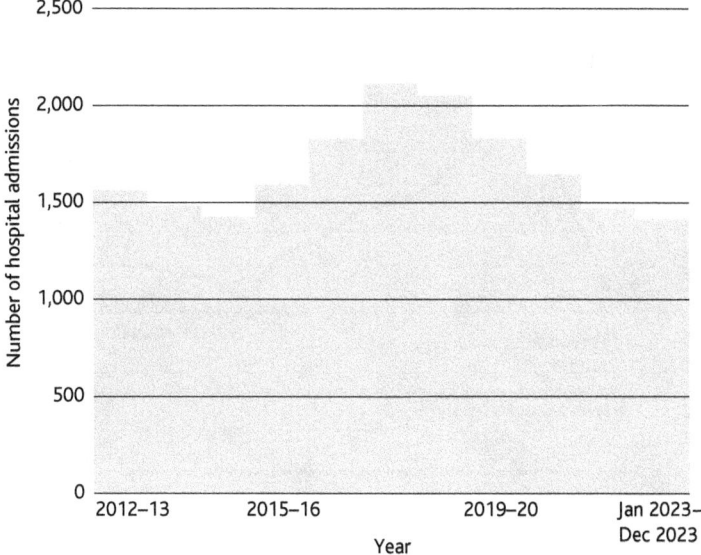

Source: NHS Digital (2023)

In keeping with the relatively pessimistic nature of public opinion on crime more generally, members of the public tend to overestimate levels of violent crime and perceive it to be getting worse, regardless of whether it is, in fact, getting better (see, for example, Office for National Statistics, 2017; Youth Endowment Fund, 2024a). For this reason, violence is arguably an issue that merits the attention of policy makers and professionals, regardless of what our best estimates suggest about trends and absolute levels of violence. Whatever the trends indicate, we must avoid complacency in the present and continue to strive towards the creation of more peaceful societies in the future.

Before we introduce the central subject of this book – the public health approach to violence prevention – we offer a note on the causes of violence. There are many excellent accounts that consider violence causation in detail (see, for example, Gilligan, 1996, 2001; Currie, 2016). Our purpose here is to review what we regard as some of the most important findings

Figure 4: Violence in London, per 1,000 people, by type, 2002–19

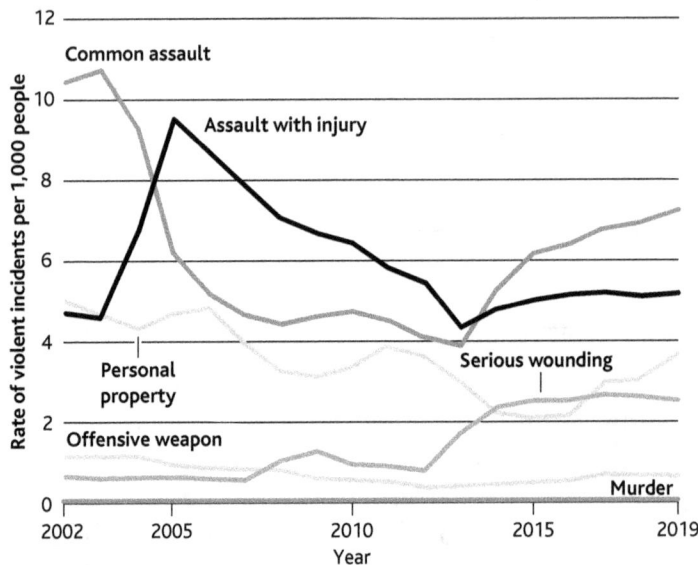

Source: Bespoke data request made to the Metropolitan Police Service

in this literature, rather than make any substantive contribution to it. This lays important foundations for the book's central topic of violence prevention.

The causes of interpersonal violence

Interpersonal violence is a complex social phenomenon. While there are many different routes into the topic, one useful starting point is the distinction between root and direct causes (Roach and Pease, 2013, pp 75–6). Sometimes these are referred to as 'distal/developmental' and 'proximate' causes respectively.

Root causes

Beginning with root causes, these sit at the back of the causal chain and include factors such as poverty, inequality, exposure to domestic violence, and access to decent housing and employment. Of note, a recently expanding literature has examined the connection between 'adverse childhood experiences' (ACEs), trauma, and violence. ACEs include factors such as being verbally, physically, or sexually abused, and living in a home where adults have a mental illness or abuse drugs or alcohol. A study examining the links between ACEs, trauma, and violence concluded that violence perpetration was more than five times higher for those who had experienced four or more ACEs compared with those who had experienced no ACEs (Bellis et al, 2014, p 4). This was explained on the basis that 'early life trauma can lead to structural and functional changes in the brain and its stress regulatory systems, which affect factors such as emotional regulation and fear response, and this may predispose individuals to HHBs [health-harming behaviours, including violence]' (Bellis et al, 2014, p 6). In a similar vein, Gray et al (2023) highlight the links between ACEs, trauma, and violent behaviour, highlighting the adverse impact that ACEs can have on children and young people's minds, bodies, and need for belonging.

Lending some support to these findings, research in the field of developmental criminology has identified a series of 'risk' and 'protective' factors, many of which might be considered root causes. These factors increase or decrease the propensity of violence and other forms of harmful behaviour, and span:

- early childhood, including exposure to domestic violence, neglect, and harsh parenting;
- adolescence, including peer influence and school attachment;
- adulthood, including marriage and unemployment (see Sampson and Laub, 1993; Loeber and Stouthamer-Loeber, 1998; Farrington, 2005).

While risk factors might correlate with violence, the extent to which these factors have a causal relationship with violence is less straightforward (Farrington, 2000). In addition, some scholars have critiqued this way of making sense of crime and violence, arguing that it can lead to the stigmatisation and marginalisation of already vulnerable groups (Armstrong, 2004; Goddard, 2014).

Recent research has also considered the role of biological factors, including genetics, neurochemistry, and brain structure and function (Raine, 2019; Pardini et al, 2014). Raine (2013), for example, argues that damage to the prefrontal cortex – which, among other things, is responsible for inhibiting aggressive impulses – can predispose individuals to violent behaviour, especially when combined with environmental stressors such as child abuse.

Direct causes

In contrast to root causes, direct causes are those that trigger, or directly relate to, a specific incident of violence in the 'here and now' (Roach and Pease, 2013, p 75). These include weapon possession, threats, disrespect, instrumental motivations (for example, immediate financial gain), and alcohol use. Adopting a micro-sociological analysis, Collins (2008) has argued that committing interpersonal violence is hard and relatively rare. He provides an extensive analysis of situational factors, such as emotional energy and the role of bystanders, which make the commission of violence possible under certain circumstances.

Explanations of violence causation might focus on root causes, direct causes, or attempt to make sense of the complex relations between the two.

The ecological framework

Another potential lens has been developed by the World Health Organization (WHO) (World Health Organization, no date), which frames violence as an outcome of factors operating at four different levels of an 'ecological framework': the societal, the community, the relational, and the individual (see Figure 5).

The people, neighbourhoods, and communities most affected by violence are typically those that experience a complex interweaving of factors across all four levels. By way of example, it is well established that levels of poverty and inequality are closely linked to levels of alcohol and substance abuse, both of which have different causal pathways to violence (Room, 2005).

While the ecological model identifies factors associated with violence, it does not explain the reasons for these associations. James Gilligan, an American prison psychiatrist and researcher, has

Figure 5: An ecological framework for understanding the factors linked to violence

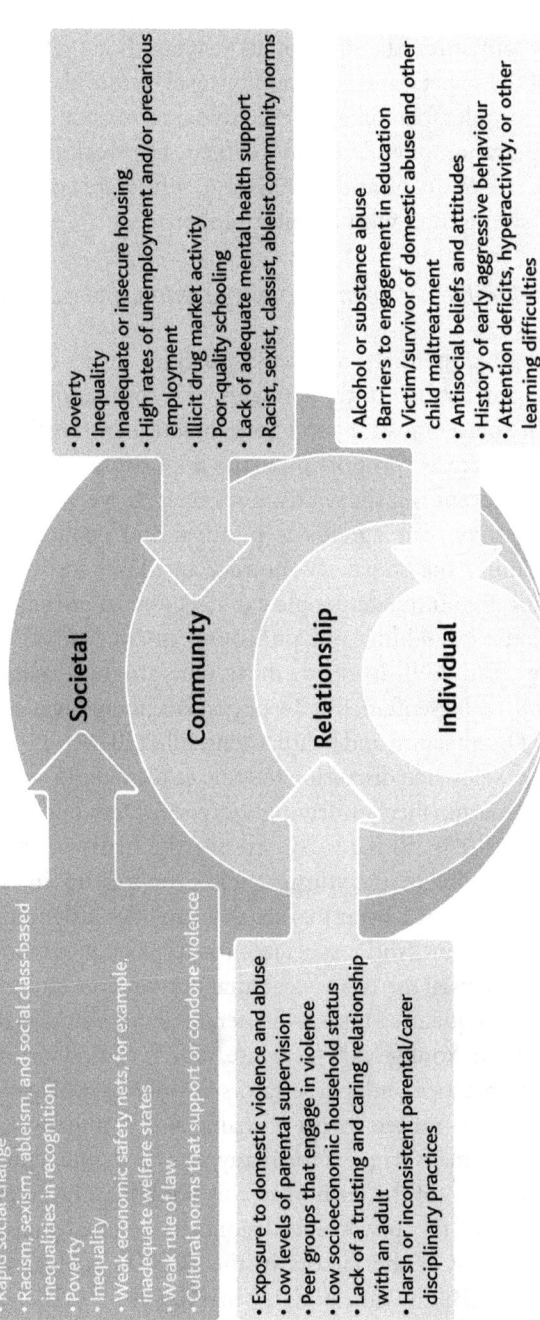

Source: Fraser and Irwin-Rogers (2021), adapted from World Health Organization (no date)

produced a highly influential account of violence that has helped advance our understanding of its drivers. For Gilligan (1996), many of the societal and community-level factors identified earlier generate intolerable forms of psychological tension, which make the perpetration of violence more likely. His work focuses on the prominence of shame and humiliation, which are common in the lives of young men who commit violence.

The relationship between shame, mattering, and violence

Gilligan suggests that societies with high levels of inequality, poverty, patriarchal cultural norms, discrimination, and other forms of social injustice tend to generate high levels of shame among a significant proportion of the population. With regards to violence prevention, then, he argues that: 'If we wish to prevent violence, then, our agenda is political and economic reform … reforming the social, economic, and legal institutions that systematically humiliate people can do more to prevent violence than all the preaching and punishing in the world' (Gilligan, 1996, pp 236, 239). In short, those who are most marginalised, powerless, and disenfranchised – or perceive themselves to be – feel a sense of humiliation and belittlement. Ellis (2016, p 110) captures this point well when discussing the role of masculinity and 'shame-inducing marginality' in driving violence. Drawing on Winlow and Hall (2013), Ellis (2016) stresses the crisis of masculinity experienced by many young men growing up in a weakly regulated capitalist labour market that provides little opportunity for secure, decent, and respectable forms of employment. Other scholars have used the term 'structural humiliation' to denote how structural inequalities tend to generate acute emotional distress (Sayer, 2005; Young, 2007; White, 2013). Based on extensive psychiatric practice with perpetrators of violence, Gilligan suggests that these deep-rooted forms of shame and humiliation, in turn, serve as proximate triggers for many acts of serious violence.

Similarly, two of the authors of this book have highlighted the importance of the psychosocial concept of 'mattering', which connects many of the factors in the WHO's ecological model of violence (Billingham and Irwin-Rogers, 2022). Mattering is made up of two components. The first is a feeling of social significance, built on trusting and meaningful relationships that help people to recognise their value to others. The second is a feeling of agency – that a person can make a difference in the world and experience a degree of control and power in their lives (as opposed to feeling diminished and powerless). Factors such as inequality, poverty, inadequate housing, exclusionary forms of education, and high rates of precarious employment can serve to undermine young people's sense of mattering, and the cumulative effects of these factors from the earliest years of life can leave a young person feeling insignificant and powerless (Flett, 2018).

A lack of mattering can make the perpetration of violence more likely for several reasons. First, if a young person feels a shameful or humiliating sense of insignificance and powerlessness, their behaviour is likely to be more volatile in the face of interpersonal disrespect than someone with a secure sense of their own significance and power. Young people who lack a firm sense of mattering are more likely to experience insults or disrespect as fundamental threats to their self-identity, which can result in highly emotional and physically violent responses. Second, young people who feel that they do not matter are far more likely to end up in situations where they are more exposed to the risk of serious violence. For example, young people who perceive themselves to be lacking in social significance are much more likely than their peers to become gang-involved as a route to achieving recognition and power, or due to heightened vulnerability to exploitation (Billingham and Irwin-Rogers, 2022). In turn, gang involvement entails a higher risk of conflict with other groups of young people, as well as increased exposure to the violence inherent in the operation of illicit drug markets (Harding, 2014; Fraser, 2017; Irwin-Rogers, 2019; McLean, 2019; Spicer et al, 2020).

In summary, the question of what causes violence is complex, with numerous causal factors operating at different levels. The WHO's ecological model provides a useful orienting device because it draws attention to factors that sit at four levels, ranging from the societal to the individual. Meanwhile, the work of Gilligan (1996) and others has aided our understanding of how factors at these different levels are connected – showing, for instance, how societal and community-level factors can generate psychological tensions within individuals, which make violent behaviour more likely. Effective violence prevention strategies, then – including the public health approach to violence prevention – are likely to be those that address drivers of violence operating at all four levels of the ecological model.

The public health approach to violence prevention

There are many references throughout this book to the public health approach to violence prevention. While the roots of this approach date back a number of decades, it is only in recent years that it has received considerable policy traction in England and Wales. With substantial confusion over its meaning and uncertainty regarding its future, this book provides a timely discussion of the public health approach's current limitations as well as the potential it still holds, if it were to be conceptualised and implemented differently. When the term is used – whether by politicians, journalists, professionals, or academics – it often lacks sufficient explanation. In Part I of this book, we will provide a short history of the public health approach to violence prevention. For now, we offer a brief insight into what we regard as the limitations of current interpretations of the public health approach, before proposing some refinements based on a 'Four Is' framework.

The limitations of existing interpretations of the public health approach

When explicit references to the public health approach to violence prevention began to appear in the US in the 1980s, the central argument being made was that significant and longlasting violence prevention could not be achieved through law enforcement alone (US Department of Health and Human Services, 1986). From this starting point, a plurality of voices emerged on how a public health approach to violence prevention might develop.

Three core elements are often associated with the public health approach to violence prevention:

- **ecology of causes – 'the what':** recognising that violence is driven not by any single factor, but by a multitude of factors

operating at the societal, community, relational, and individual levels (World Health Organization, no date; see Figure 5);
- **stages of prevention – 'the when':** ensuring that efforts to prevent violence involve an appropriate balance of work at the primary level (before it occurs), secondary level (immediate responses to violence, such as pre-hospital care and emergency services), and tertiary level (long-term care in the wake of violence, such as rehabilitation and reintegration) (Krug et al, 2002, p 15);
- **model of implementation – 'the how':** following the World Health Organization's (no date) four-step model: (i) defining and mapping the problem of violence; (ii) identifying the causes of violence; (iii) designing, implementing, and evaluating interventions to find out what works to prevent violence; and (iv) embedding and scaling up interventions that work.

In England and Wales today, while policy makers have ostensibly committed to the public health approach to violence prevention and these core elements, in practice, we see something more partial and limited. Specifically – as we shall see throughout this book – there is serious neglect of societal and community-level drivers of violence, accompanied by a lack of primary prevention. Current efforts to prevent violence focus predominantly on secondary and tertiary prevention, typically through multi-agency working and programmatic interventions that attempt to change individual attitudes and behaviour (Riemann, 2019). In a recent rapid review of public health approaches, Walsh and colleagues (2023, p 25) concluded that 'central to PH–VP [public health approach to violence prevention] is choosing and facilitating programmes' – programmes that almost invariably operate at a local level and target those deemed most 'at risk' of violence.

To fully realise the potential of the public health approach, it must be understood and applied holistically, from hyper-local interventions in certain communities, to policy change at the highest levels of government. To encourage a shift away from the currently narrow and limited violence prevention strategy that we see in England and Wales, we promote the use of a 'Four Is' framework.

Advancing the public health approach using the 'Four Is' framework

The 'Four Is' framework was developed by Billingham as part of the 'Public Health, Youth and Violence Reduction' (PHYVR) project. It serves to highlight the limitations that we saw with the existing public health approach to violence prevention in England and Wales, and provides an indication of how its scope could be broadened. The framework is based on the idea that violence prevention activity can and should take place at different levels, from the macro to the micro (see Figure 6).

At the macro level, efforts to prevent violence might include government policies that attempt to address various societal inequalities, including inequalities in wealth, income, opportunity, recognition, power, and exposure to different forms of risk (for example, homelessness, unemployment, ill health, and so on). Remaining at the macro level, violence prevention activities might also focus on improving key societal institutions, services, and social infrastructure across England and Wales, such as schools, social care, youth justice, family services, and community leisure facilities, all of which can play a pivotal role in shaping the quality of children and young people's lives.

At a more local (or micro) level, efforts to reduce violence might involve the delivery of a range of interventions or programmes, including cognitive behavioural therapy, focused deterrence, and sports programmes. Finally, at the extreme micro end of the framework, we have the individual interactions and relationships that young people have with their families and communities, and with professionals. These interactions and relationships have the greatest direct influence on children and young people, and are crucial in

Figure 6: The Four Is framework

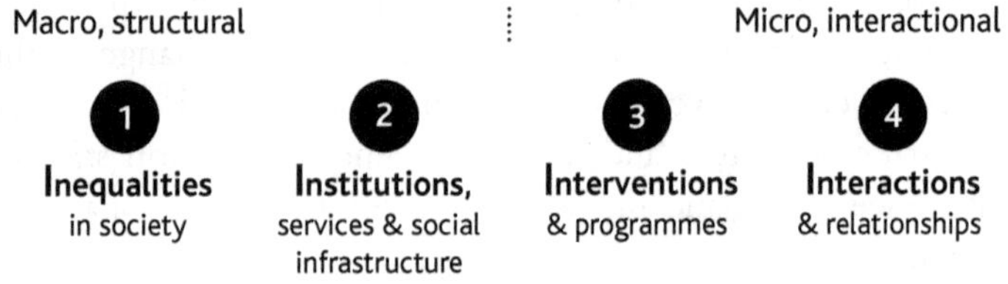

Macro, structural · · · · · Micro, interactional

1 **Inequalities** in society

2 **Institutions,** services & social infrastructure

3 **Interventions** & programmes

4 **Interactions** & relationships

shaping their day-to-day lives. As we will explore further throughout this book, these interactions and relationships are also influenced in various ways by the other three levels of the Four Is framework.

To summarise, our core argument is that the public health approach to violence prevention is best conceptualised in broad terms, encapsulating many of the sentiments and ideas initially mooted at the US Surgeon General's seminal workshop on violence and public health in 1985 (US Department of Health and Human Services, 1986, discussed in more detail in Chapter 1). As time has passed, there appears to have been an unhelpful narrowing of the nature and scope of the public health approach – in part a consequence of people and groups attempting to put principles into practice in their specific domains of authority and expertise, operating within the prevailing policy paradigms of particular jurisdictions. Our primary aim is to rejuvenate the essence of a holistic public health approach to violence prevention, and explain what this might look like in policy and practice.

Researching the public health approach to violence prevention

This book is based on a three-year project funded by the ESRC, entitled 'Public Health, Youth and Violence Reduction' (PHYVR). The study, which took place between January 2021 and January 2024, examined public health approaches to violence prevention in Scotland, England, and Wales. It attempted to make sense of the significant decline in violence seen in Scotland between the years 2006–15, and to consider the extent to which lessons might be drawn from the Scottish experience and applied elsewhere. The study also sought to examine the extent to which a public health approach appeared to be emerging in England and Wales, and the implications of recent policy shifts.

The project team generated and collected data from four main sources.

Interviews and focus groups

Interviews were conducted with a total of 189 people across Scotland, England, and Wales.[3] This included 109 participants who held relatively senior positions at the level of policy and practice, such as policy makers in Holyrood and Westminster (senior civil servants and current and former ministers), and strategic leads and managers across policing, youth justice, health, education, and social care. At a community level, the team conducted area-based case studies in communities affected by violence in Glasgow and London, which involved 43 interviews with community leaders and youth practitioners, as well as a period of participant observation with community-based youth organisations. The study also involved focus groups and interviews with 37 children and young people living in communities affected by violence. All interviews adopted a semi-structured approach, with interview schedules containing questions about the perceived nature of violence in local communities and interviewees' perceptions of violence prevention efforts. In each interview, we provided space for the discussion to move in different directions, depending on participants' responses.

For the purpose of this book, 20 interviews in particular are worth noting: those conducted with all 20 of the regional Violence Reduction Units (VRUs) in England and Wales. VRUs will be introduced and discussed at length in the following chapters. Here, it is enough to note that VRUs were established across different regions in England and Wales between 2018 and 2021, largely in an attempt to replicate the perceived success of the Scottish VRU in reducing violence during the preceding decade. The vast majority of interview extracts in Part II were taken from our interviews with VRU directors. Typically, these interviews were conducted one-to-one with the director of the VRU, but in some cases, additional VRU team members joined at a director's request. The interviews followed a similar structure, beginning with discussions of the emergence and early work of the VRU, proceeding to consider how the VRU's work had evolved over time, and finishing by reflecting on directors' hopes and visions for the future. In among these discussions, directors were commonly asked to comment on the relationship between the work of the VRU and other partner agencies, their understanding of the concept of the 'public health approach' and its implications, and the major challenges and barriers that their VRUs had already faced and were facing in the years ahead.

Introduction

With a small number of exceptions, our interviews were conducted and recorded online. Interview recordings were transcribed by a professional transcription service, and then uploaded to the software package NVivo. While some interviewees waived their right to anonymity, many others did not. Although much of the content of our conversations was relatively uncontroversial and not of a particularly sensitive nature, at times, interviews touched on issues that interviewees may have felt more comfortable talking about in a frank and open way under conditions of anonymity. To avoid a situation in which some interview extracts were attributed to a particular interviewee while others were not, we decided to anonymise all extracts contained in this book for consistency.

Adaptive theory was used to analyse the transcripts – an 'accretive' method of analysis, which involves approaching the data with some prior conceptual framework(s) in mind but being open to amending them subject to what the researcher perceives the data to be 'saying' (see Layder, 1998, p 156). Four members of the PHYVR team were involved in the coding process, meeting periodically to discuss coded transcripts and potential improvements to the emergent coding frameworks. In relation to the VRU transcripts in particular, one member of the team analysed the full set initially, before sharing six coded transcripts with three other members of the PHYVR team. Subsequent group discussions of the coded transcripts enabled the initial team member to check their understanding of the data, and refine the conceptual categories used to make sense of it.

Documentary analysis

A systematic and comprehensive documentary analysis examined the emergence and development of public health approaches to violence prevention in Scotland, England, and Wales. The sources covered by the analysis included policy documents, legislation, official statements, public and third sector reports, and outputs from mainstream and social media. In Scotland, the documentary analysis extended back to Scotland's Social Work (Scotland) Act 1968, while in England and Wales the starting point was the coming to power of New Labour in 1997.

Police-recorded crime data

To examine trends in different types of violence over time, police-recorded crime data were examined for Scotland, England, and Wales over a 20-year period, focusing on Glasgow and London in particular. Bespoke requests were made to Police Scotland and the London Metropolitan Police for granular data that were not otherwise publicly available. Secondary data on violence trends, which used modelling techniques to offer a fine-grained analysis of recorded violence, were used to triangulate emergent findings from the qualitative interviews. Specific methods included temporal and spatial analysis, including growth mixture modelling, to identify changing trajectories of violence (as used by Bannister et al, 2017; McVie et al, 2020).

Workshops with regional VRUs

Two online workshops were held with all 20 directors of the regional VRUs in England and Wales to explore and scrutinise key themes emerging from our semi-structured interviews. Each of these workshops lasted for around three hours and consisted of brief presentations of key themes from the PHYVR team, followed by free-flowing comments and feedback. Subsequently, we held a full-day face-to-face workshop in London, to which all VRU directors and members of their teams were invited; 46 people attended in total. Key topics of discussion included the implementation of the Serious Violence Duty, engagement with communities and young people, and what makes for an effective VRU.

Ethics

The project obtained ethical approval from the University of Glasgow's College Research Ethics Committee (Application No: 400200136). In addition, a Data Protection Impact Assessment (DPIA) was conducted to ensure compliance with GDPR. This involved detailing the project's data processing activities, identifying potential risks and outlining corresponding mitigation strategies. The PHYVR team developed project information sheets and privacy notices, which were provided to all participants prior to data collection. Prior to each interview and focus group, researchers ensured there was sufficient time for participants to ask questions and express any concerns about the research process.

As noted earlier, participants were offered the choice of their data being anonymised or opting out of anonymisation. For participants whose roles made anonymisation unfeasible – such as high-profile public figures – the implications of non-anonymity were discussed in detail before participation. If data required anonymisation, then transcripts were reviewed and edited to include pseudonyms and remove potential identifiers. All participants provided written informed consent and were informed of their right to withdraw their data up to 12 months following their participation. All data were securely stored on encrypted, password-protected University of Glasgow servers.

Summary

A significant amount of qualitative and quantitative data has been generated and collected as part of the PHYVR project. Taken together, and considered alongside the extant literature, these data provide solid foundations for each part of the book as outlined in the following section.

Structure and style

A key source of inspiration orienting this study has been the work of economic geographer, Bent Flyvbjerg. In *Making Social Science Matter*, Flyvbjerg (2001) questions the wisdom of attempting to develop predictive theory about the social world. He regards this as a flawed quest to emulate the success of the natural sciences, and instead argues that the contextualised nature of all social action makes it more fruitful to focus on the particular and the concrete. Flyvbjerg calls for researchers to address the following three key questions:

- Where are we going?
- Is this desirable?
- What should be done?

In the spirit of these questions, this book explores:

- where we are going in the area of violence prevention in England and Wales;
- if this direction of travel is desirable;
- what should be done in the years ahead.

More specifically, it seeks to assess the past, present, and future of the public health approach to violence prevention. When properly conceptualised, and implemented with care and commitment, this approach has the potential to bring about safe and secure societies for children, young people and adults alike.

We have divided the book into three parts.

Part I: A short history of the public health approach to violence prevention

The first part of the book, comprising Chapters 1 and 2, addresses the following two questions:

- What are the origins of the public health approach to violence prevention and how did it develop over time?
- What are the main strengths and limitations associated with the way the public health approach is currently conceptualised and implemented?

Here, we provide a short history of the public health approach to violence prevention in England and Wales, with some consideration of the influence of other jurisdictions including the US and Scotland. Chapter 1 describes the long-term development of the public health approach since the 1980s. Chapter 2 focuses more specifically on the period 2018–23 in England and Wales, a crucial few years during which the UK government publicly stated its intention to adopt a public health approach to violence prevention, and instigated a range of measures to bring it to life.

Part II: Violence Reduction Units

The second part of the book, comprising Chapters 3 and 4, addresses the following two questions:

- What role do VRUs play in advancing the public health approach?
- What are the main opportunities and challenges facing VRUs?

This part of the book presents key findings from our interviews with VRU directors and other team members across the VRU network to explore the stories of these units, including the main challenges and opportunities they have faced during their early years. While VRU directors and members of their teams are not the only important sources of information when it comes to understanding the work of VRUs, their leadership roles mean they are well placed to offer informed reflections on the nature and value of VRUs' work to date. They are also in a good position to provide reflections on how best VRUs can be taken forward in the years ahead, if they are to have the greatest chance of success in preventing serious violence between young people.

Part III: Looking ahead

The final part of the book, comprising Chapter 5, considers the following questions:

- How can a truly holistic public health approach to violence prevention be conceptualised?
- What steps are needed to turn this vision into reality in England and Wales?

Here, we reflect on recent violence prevention initiatives in England and Wales. This part of the book promotes a vision of a truly holistic public health approach to violence prevention, considering the potential implications of a 'Four Is' framework. In short, this entails a comprehensive response to violence that requires action being taken at the levels of inequalities, institutions, interventions, and interactions.

While each part of the book has a distinct focus, there are also important connections between them. For example, Part I's short history of the public health approach to violence prevention provides useful context for the discussion of VRUs' emergence and ongoing work in Part II. VRUs have been tasked with advancing the public health approach across regions in England and Wales with the highest rates of violence, and their scope and functions cannot be fully understood unless they are embedded within a broader understanding of how work around violence prevention has unfolded in recent years. Equally, when we address Part III's guiding question, 'Where should we go from here?', our argument is underpinned by material in Parts I and II.

As the outline we have given suggests, the remainder of the book adopts a broadly chronological structure. Reflecting the book's subtitle, Part I concerns the past, Part II the present, and Part III the future. Chapter 1 begins this journey by taking us back to the early roots of the public health approach to violence prevention.

PART I

A short history of the public health approach to violence prevention

PART I

A short history of the numerical approaches to solute geochemistry prediction

1

Roots and shoots of the public health approach to violence prevention

The public health approach to violence prevention was formally adopted first as regional policy in London in 2018, and then as national policy in England and Wales in 2019. During this period, serious violence in England and Wales was on the rise. In Scotland, by contrast, rates of violence were broadly stable and at their lowest levels of the 21st century. As London Mayor, Sadiq Khan, and United Kingdom (UK) Prime Minister, Theresa May, made clear at the time, their decisions to pursue a public health approach were inspired by the perceived success of violence reduction in Scotland (Mayor of London, 2018; Gourtsoyannis, 2019; Home Office, 2019h).

This chapter examines the historical background to these decisions, exploring how the public health approach emerged and developed in policy and practice, first in Scotland and later in England and Wales. To set the longer-term historical context, we consider the history of youth justice in Scotland from the early post-war period. Some of the philosophical principles associated with Scotland's contemporary public health approach to violence prevention are clearly present in this historical account. Next, we discuss the establishment of the Scottish Violence Reduction Unit (VRU), and the influence of the World Health Organization (WHO) and United States (US)-based public health initiatives on subsequent developments in Scotland. Understanding Scotland's journey towards a public health approach to violence prevention is important, because events in Scotland came to play a key role in shaping the public health approach to violence prevention south of the border.

The final section of the chapter turns to England and Wales and their long-term trajectory of youth justice. This section takes us up to 2018 and the point at which the public health approach to violence prevention was formally adopted in London. Chapter 2 then provides a detailed examination of how the public health approach to violence prevention emerged, first in London and later across England and Wales, and then developed over the period 2018–23. Before turning our attention to Scotland, this chapter begins by looking at the some of the earliest roots of public health approaches, which emerged in the US in the 1980s.

Early roots of the public health approach to violence prevention

Contemporary public health approaches to violence prevention have their origins in the 1980s, when an influential report by the US Department of Health and Human Services (1986) was produced following a workshop on 'violence and public health' organised by the US Surgeon General. The report contained a series of papers from a diverse group of experts in the field of violence prevention, all of whom recognised the limitations of relying solely on law enforcement to prevent interpersonal violence.

The papers varied in their scope and focus, but, taken together, they covered many of the elements that are today recognised as falling under the banner of a public health approach to violence prevention. One contributor, for example, argued that violence prevention should involve the consideration of a broad spectrum of social issues, including, but not limited to, the provision of 'better schools, safer housing, [and] more jobs for disadvantaged youngsters' (US Department of Health and Human Services, 1986, p 47). Another contributor emphasised that 'surveillance is essential … we must define all aspects of the problem, collect relevant and accurate data, analyse that data in order to define interventions, and measure the impact of those interventions' (US Department of Health and Human Services,

1986, p 20). Specifically on the issue of assault and homicide, the report recommended that 'a full employment policy should be developed and implemented for the nation', that there should be an 'aggressive policy to reduce racial discrimination and sexism', and that 'health care providers, criminal justice agencies, schools and social service agencies should communicate and cooperate to a greater extent in order to improve the identification and treatment of – and early intervention for – high-risk individuals' (US Department of Health and Human Services, 1986, pp 52–3).

Rather than laying out in clear and exclusive terms what a public health approach to violence prevention ought to look like, the report presented a plurality of voices on the topic of violence prevention. Each of these voices stressed different features of what they regarded to be potentially effective approaches to preventing violence. As we shall see throughout Part I, echoes of these early voices can be found in many subsequent manifestations of the public health approach to violence prevention across a number of jurisdictions.

The origins and development of Scotland's public health approach

Youth (juvenile) justice

While Scotland fell under the general governance of the UK Parliament until the Scotland Act 1998 established the now devolved Scottish Parliament, the 1707 Acts of Union preserved Scotland's distinctive legal system. This meant that Scotland's youth justice system evolved separately to that in England and Wales, diverging in important ways at different points in history (McVie, 2017). The greatest point of divergence, and the one most critical to underpinning a public health approach in Scotland, was sparked by the Kilbrandon Report (1964), which set out the blueprint for a new system of youth justice predicated on the 'needs' rather than the 'deeds' of children and young people. Enshrined in the Social Work (Scotland) Act 1968, almost all of the recommendations from the Kilbrandon Report were implemented – including the abolition of youth courts – and a new Children's Hearings System came into being in 1971. The Hearings System, which 'aimed at early and minimal intervention' (McAra, 2017, p 952) was designed to give children and young people, and the adults working with them, the chance to discuss their life circumstances, and to make legally binding decisions about any necessary social or educational support. Still in operation today, Children's Hearings can be held in response both to child protection concerns and to a child's law-breaking behaviour, as they are arranged on the premise that the underlying needs of the child are paramount. For the most part, the Hearings System has been regarded as more welfare-oriented, more child-friendly, and less punitive than youth justice arrangements south of the border (Hothersall, 2012).

While the 1968 Act set Scottish youth justice on a very different path from that in England and Wales in the latter decades of the 20th century, a shift back towards policy convergence occurred briefly in the early 21st century. Following the opening of the Scottish Parliament in 1999, the new political regime sought to assert its authority over a range of policy domains, including youth justice. An Advisory Group on Youth Crime was appointed and a report quickly published entitled *It's a Criminal Waste: Stop youth crime now* (Scottish Executive, 2000). A subsequent Action Plan highlighted the need to increase public confidence in youth justice, place a greater focus on victims, and ease the transition between youth and adult justice systems. Taking inspiration from its neighbours south of the border, where the New Labour government at Westminster had pledged to be 'tough on crime, tough on the causes of crime' (1997), the government in Scotland introduced a raft of new legislation, including the Anti-Social Behaviour (Scotland) Act 2004, which heralded a more punitive approach to dealing with young people. As part of the experiment, a new system of 'fast-track' Hearings was introduced in a number of pilot areas in 2005, with the aim of dealing more quickly, cheaply, and effectively with those involved in persistent offending. Scotland's flirtation with penal populism was, however, just that – a flirtation that ended in failure after research demonstrated that the fast-track Hearings, far from achieving appreciable reductions in offending and saving money, were making existing problems worse (Hill et al, 2005). The fast-track Hearings were hastily abandoned, and Scotland's system of youth justice reverted to its original form.

Getting it Right for Every Child

This point in Scotland's history marks a crucial step in the development of social policy concerning children and young people. From the ashes of the failed punitive policies introduced by the Scottish Executive, a new policy document emerged in 2006 entitled *Getting it Right for Every Child* (GIRFEC) (Scottish Executive, 2006). Emanating from a review of the Hearings system, GIRFEC harked back to the principles espoused by the Kilbrandon Report and focused on improving children's wellbeing in Scotland. GIRFEC was described by one group of commentators as a 'landmark policy framework ... representing an aspirational and transformational change agenda in terms of promoting well-being and embodying new working practices' (Coles et al, 2016, p 335). It had two distinguishing characteristics: first, it embodied a holistic approach to understanding children's needs, and contained an aspirational commitment to all Scotland's children; and, second, it proposed a 'whole policy/whole country implementation and national transformational change agenda' (Coles et al, 2016, p 335).

In addition to its core emphasis on children's wellbeing, GIRFEC's principles included: 'taking a whole child approach', 'co-ordinating help', and 'building a competent workforce' in order to promote such principles (Scottish Executive, 2006). Not only did GIRFEC reflect the Kilbrandon principles that had underpinned the establishment of the Children's Hearings System in 1971, but it also aligned with the more recently implemented United Nations Convention on the Rights of the Child, which came into force in 1992. The new framework's primary focus was on matters such as children's wellbeing and equality, directing attention away from offending, and affirming care over control. It also deliberately avoided the more punitive rhetoric that had characterised the politics of youth offending in Scotland earlier in the century, and which was prominent in many other jurisdictions at the time, including England and Wales.

In 2007, the arrival in power of a new Scottish National Party (SNP)-led government helped herald what has been portrayed as a new 'progressive era' in responses to youth offending in Scotland (McAra and McVie, 2018). Published in 2008, *Preventing Offending by Young People: A framework for action* set out the new government's strategy for the prevention of offending (Scottish Government, 2008c). In this context, and alongside GIRFEC and its Early Years Framework (an approach to maximising quality of life from pre-birth to age eight), it instituted a pilot programme aimed at trialling a new 'whole-system approach' to youth offending. Among other things, this involved a commitment to diversion and to what it referred to as 'early and effective intervention' (Scottish Government, 2008c). Underpinned by findings from the Edinburgh Study of Youth Transitions and Crime (McAra and McVie, 2010b), the whole-system approach was rolled out to all 32 local authorities across Scotland from 2011 (Lightowler et al, 2014).

The establishment of the Scottish VRU

These changes to the youth justice system represent a significant backdrop to the development of a public health approach in Scotland as they align with contemporaneous changes to the development of new strategies for reducing violence. In the year preceding the publication of GIRFEC in 2006, two important articles about levels of violence in Scotland appeared in the media. The first, which appeared on the BBC News website on 18 September 2005, alleged that a United Nations report had named Scotland as 'the most violent country in the developed world' (BBC News, 2005). Based on a telephone survey across 21 countries, the report was said to have declared that 'Scots were almost three times as likely to be assaulted as Americans', and that the rate of violence in Scotland 'dwarfs that of other developed nations such as Japan, where people are 30 times less likely to be attacked' (BBC News, 2005). Just days later, on 26 September 2005, *The Guardian* newspaper published a second article entitled 'Scotland has second highest murder rate in Europe' (Seenan, 2005). Allegedly based on a WHO study, involving 21 countries from Western Europe, Scotland was said to have a rate of homicide that was three times higher than that in England and Wales, the second highest only to Finland. The *Guardian* article also alleged that a forthcoming study from the University of California would 'claim Scotland has a higher homicide rate than America,

Israel, Uzbekistan, Chile and Uruguay' (Seenan, 2005). These articles are problematic, for a number of reasons: first, it is now impossible to track down the two reports on which these claims were made; second, the reported differences in violence rates between countries were often marginal and it is not clear that they were tested for statistical significance; and, third, some of these claims were subsequently discredited (for example, a correction published by *The Guardian* on 24 October 2005 clarified that the murder rate for the US was actually more than double that for Scotland). Nevertheless, the ramifications of these two articles were deep and long lasting.

One of the most notable actions taken in response to these damning reports was the creation of a VRU by the-then Strathclyde Police Force, the largest of Scotland's eight forces at the time. The Force's chief, Sir Willie Rae, tasked two people – Detective Superintendent, John Carnochan, and principal analyst, Karyn McCluskey – with establishing a small team to work on developing a new approach to the problem of violence. Originally focused only on Glasgow, the work of the VRU was expanded in 2006 to include the whole of Scotland (henceforth the Scottish VRU), now with the financial support and backing of the Scottish government. The Scottish VRU continued to sit within Strathclyde Police, and undertook a range of enforcement initiatives, such as expansive weapons-sweeps and mass stop and search. Over time, however, it came to embrace an approach that emphasised the importance of prevention and early support to young people at risk of violence, recognising that enforcement alone could not produce substantial and long-lasting reductions in violent behaviour. The synergies with what was happening more broadly in Scottish youth justice, described earlier, were clear.

Inspiration and influence from the WHO and the US

As the Scottish VRU evolved over time, the language of 'public health' increasingly came to the fore, driven in large part by the work of the WHO. In its first *World Report on Violence and Health*, published in 2002, the WHO described the problem of violence as a 'public health' issue (Krug et al, 2002). Established at a WHO meeting on violence prevention in 2004, an initiative called the Violence Prevention Alliance lent its weight to the importance of systematic data collection and the evaluation of interventions, arguing that public health approaches to violence prevention ought to follow a four-step model:

1. To define the problem through the systematic collection of information about the magnitude, scope, characteristics and consequences of violence.
2. To establish why violence occurs using research to determine the causes and correlates of violence, the factors that increase or decrease the risk for violence, and the factors that could be modified through interventions.
3. To find out what works to prevent violence by designing, implementing and evaluating interventions.
4. To implement effective and promising interventions in a wide range of settings. The effects of these interventions on risk factors and the target outcome should be monitored, and their impact and cost-effectiveness should be evaluated. (World Health Organization, no date)

One of the most common violence prevention strategies grounded in this four-step model is focused deterrence, implemented initially in the US before spreading to other countries across the world, including Scotland (Braga and Weisburd, 2015, p 58; Braga et al, 2019). A concrete manifestation of focused deterrence that came to influence the Scottish VRU was Boston's Ceasefire initiative, which involved problem-oriented policing targeting youth homicide. With research at its heart, it combined a carrot-and-stick approach by sending a clear 'zero tolerance' message to gang members about violence, combined with support from social workers, probation and parole officers, churches, and other community groups, which offered a variety of services around substance abuse, education, and employment. The project was widely credited with generating declines in homicide of over 60 per cent (Kennedy et al, 2001).

Another violence prevention initiative that came to inspire the Scottish VRU was Cure Violence (CV), which began by focusing on several US cities between 2000 and 2008 before expanding globally. CV adheres to public health principles by viewing violence as a 'communicable disease that passes from person to person when left untreated' (Butts et al, 2015, p 39). It requires the identification of those most at risk of violence and the subsequent deployment of 'violence interrupters' (often those with their own first-hand experiences of crime and violence) to intervene and prevent violent behaviour. As with Ceasefire, CV involves communicating with the targeted audience – in this case gang members known to have committed violence or to be 'at risk' of involvement in violence – through 'offender notification meetings', 'call-ins', or 'forums', in which warnings about law enforcement and punishment are delivered (Engel et al, 2013). This, combined with support and assistance for those who want to change their lifestyle, together with various forms of community engagement, constitute the core of the approach.

Following a visit by members of the Scottish VRU to the US, many features of focused deterrence found their way back to Scotland and were embedded within the country's new commitment to a public health approach to violence prevention. Inspired by Ceasefire and CV, the Scottish VRU ran its first 'call-in' in October 2008 – a meeting involving 85 gang members aged between 16 and 22, together with local community members. Each of the gang members was given a card on arrival, which had a free phone number offering a 24/7 service to anyone who wanted to leave gang-related violence behind. The key message of the day was a choice: continue with violence and expect a robust criminal justice response; or opt to leave violence behind and expect help and support to do so. It was the first of ten 'self-referral sessions' run over the next two years, attended by over 600 men and women in total.

The Scottish VRU claimed that, among those involved in the sessions, violent crime reduced by 46 per cent, gang fighting by 73 per cent and weapon carrying by 85 per cent (VRU, 2020). Broader cultural changes were also reported, including improvements in residents' assessments of their local communities and reductions in the number of people reporting feel unsafe at night. It is worth noting, however, that an external evaluation found no statistically significant effects on violence reduction, although it did record a reduction in weapon carrying (Williams et al, 2014).

In 2008, the Scottish VRU launched a ten-year strategic plan, fronted by both the Chief Constable of Strathclyde Police and the Scottish government's Justice Secretary, affirming a commitment to a public health approach and a shared national agenda (see Scottish Government, 2008b). Violence prevention was to be a national priority, with the approach combining enforcement and supportive interventions. The same year saw the publication of the *Achieving Our Potential* policy, a framework for tackling poverty and income inequality (Scottish Government, 2008a), together with an implementation plan, *Equally Well*, aimed at addressing health inequalities (Scottish Government, 2008b). The Ministerial Task Force behind these developments explicitly endorsed the WHO's public health approach to violence prevention. While acknowledging the importance of new tough measures that had been introduced, the Task Force noted that the 'long-term solution, however, depends on us looking much earlier to those interventions that are effective in stopping violent behaviour developing in the first place' (Scottish Government, 2008b, p 32).

Within a few years, reports in the press were claiming huge successes for Scotland's public health approach. In December 2011, under the striking headline, 'Karyn McCluskey: the woman who took on Glasgow's gangs', *The Guardian* went on to ask: 'She tackled Glasgow's gangs and slashed violent crime on the streets. So how did Karyn McCluskey get such startling results in a city once known as the murder capital of western Europe?' (Henley, 2011). By 2016, police-recorded crime statistics for non-sexual crimes of violence in Scotland were down by almost half (48 per cent) and the number of murders had fallen by 38 per cent (Scottish Government, 2019). These apparent falls, when set against the backdrop of the media articles based on the United Nations and WHO reports in 2005 (Seenan, 2005), led some to claim a 'Scottish miracle' (see Fraser and Gillon, 2023). Whatever the reality, such claims certainly drew attention in other jurisdictions, not least in England and Wales.

The journey toward a public health approach: England and Wales

Youth (juvenile) justice

In England and Wales, youth justice took a very different path to Scotland in the latter decades of the 20th century. By no means did this seem inevitable. With echoes of the Kilbrandon Report in Scotland, the Longford Report, published in 1964 by the Labour Party, recommended removing children from the criminal courts in England and Wales and paying greater attention to their needs (Goldson, 2020). A White Paper issued in 1965 made radical proposals to replace juvenile courts with a non-judicial family council (similar to the Children's Hearings in Scotland); however, this was subject to vigorous objection from members of the legal system who feared losing power and influence. Just a year after the Social Work (Scotland) Act 1968 was passed, the Children and Young Persons Act 1969 was introduced in England and Wales. While similar to its Scottish counterpart in that it heralded 'the triumph of "welfare" as the dominant ideology' (Blagg and Smith, 1989, p 99), the 1969 Act retained juvenile courts as the primary model for dealing with young people accused of offending. Moreover, following the election of a Conservative government in 1970, many of the proposals were never fully implemented (Harris, 1982). In contrast to the position in Scotland, therefore, youth courts in England and Wales continued to operate largely as before. Although care proceedings on the commission of an offence were made possible, such powers were used exceedingly sparingly, and the more traditional punitive disposals became increasingly prominent during the 1970s (Thorpe et al, 1980).

The failure to implement fully the provisions of the Children and Young Persons Act 1969 presaged a complex range of developments. The election of another Conservative government in 1979 on a 'law and order' manifesto, with its tough penal rhetoric, its plans for the reintroduction of detention centres with tougher regimes, and 'short, sharp, shock' sentences, led to concerns that custodial institutions would become ever-more central to youth justice (Chaney, 2015). Certainly, at a rhetorical level, and to a large extent practically, this was the culmination of a period in which the focus shifted from 'children in need' to the rediscovery of the 'deliberately depraved delinquent' and a subsequent emphasis on control (Tutt, 1981). The early 1990s then saw the emergence of a 'tough' bipartisan consensus in England and Wales (Downes and Newburn, 2022). This affected youth justice as all else, with the government announcing a range of measures – such as the introduction of secure training centres – intended to display its robust credentials (Johnstone and Bottomley, 1998).

Tough on crime, tough on the causes of crime?

Sweeping to power in 1997, the New Labour government saw youth justice as a primary focus for its reform efforts. Its initial activity came in the form of two pieces of legislation: the Crime and Disorder Act 1998 and the Youth Justice Criminal Evidence Act 1999. The 1998 Act created youth offending teams in recognition of the importance both of multi-agency working and of approaches and professions beyond criminal justice. It also encouraged earlier intervention in the lives of those 'at risk', and utilising both the increasingly influential 'what works' paradigm and the language of 'risk factors', the government introduced a range of new orders, including the Anti-Social Behaviour Order (ASBO). As was the case with penal policy more generally, New Labour placed greater emphasis on the 'tough on crime' element of their mantra than they did on tackling the causes of youth crime. Overall, they introduced more than 50 criminal justice-related bills and created over 4,000 new criminal offences during their 13 years in government. As noted earlier, this period marked significant convergence in the approach to youth justice between Scotland and England and Wales, despite the creation of a new Scottish Parliament.

The landscape in England and Wales changed markedly from 2010 onwards. This was visible in the approaches of a succession of Conservative or Conservative-led governments, and in the 'austerity' politics that were ushered in during the decade or so following the 2008 financial crash. There were huge budget cuts, affecting the police most obviously, and what turned out to be a hugely costly and failed experiment in the marketisation of probation services. Where young people were concerned, there was a brief and initial flirtation with the promise of a more inclusive and less hostile approach to their offending. As is so often the case with penal policy, however, it is unexpected events, most usually scandal, that sway governments into modifying their intended course of action.

Arguably the most significant factor that influenced the government's approach in this period was the riots in England in August 2011. Occurring relatively early in the life of a new Conservative–Liberal Democrat coalition government, the riots lasted for four days, resulting in several deaths, hundreds of injuries, and vast negative economic consequences. The riots also precipitated an immediate and harsh penal reaction. The police recorded over 5,000 criminal offences relating to the riots and within three months almost 2,000 people had appeared in court. There were close to 850 people in prison by the end of September 2011 due to riot-related offences, many in young offender institutions.

The riots drew attention to the often-parlous state of relations between many young people, particularly Black young people, and the police, to the discriminatory and sometimes abusive use of stop-and-search powers, and to the decreasing life chances and opportunities that many of those involved in the riots felt characterised their futures (Newburn et al, 2016a, 2016b). Although evidence was all but non-existent, the riots resulted in a range of political claims about the role of gangs in the disorder, with the Home Secretary, in a foreword to the government's major report on the subject, noting that '[o]ne thing that the riots in August did do was to bring home to the entire country just how serious a problem gang and youth violence has now become' (HM Government, 2011, p 3).

In contrast to the punitive rhetoric and practice engendered by the riots, the coalition and post-coalition governments' commitment to reducing the use of youth custody remained in place and was successful. Beginning around 2008, the next eight years saw the use of youth imprisonment drop by two thirds (HM Prison and Probation Service, 2024). In parallel, the number of young people entering the criminal justice system for the first time dropped by at least the same amount. A range of influences can be identified, from the potential diversionary consequences of the restorative justice-influenced referral orders from around 2001 onwards, to a contraction in police activity (Roberts et al, 2019).

In 2015, Charlie Taylor, later to become Chair of the Youth Justice Board, was asked to undertake a review of youth justice. In his report, Taylor (2016) called for a radical overhaul of the system such that young people were to be treated as 'children first and offenders second'. Offenders, he went on, would be:

> held to account for their offending, but with an understanding that the most effective way to achieve change will often be by improving their education, their health, their welfare, and by helping them to draw on their own strengths and resources ... In this reformed system there will be widespread recognition from the police and the courts that youth offending should be dealt with at the lowest possible level, avoiding the unnecessary escalation that will bring children further into the system and damage their life prospects. (Taylor, 2016, p 48)

There was some cross-border influence here, as the 'children first, offenders second' approach drew considerable inspiration from developments that had been emerging in Wales, and was not dissimilar to the already well-established Children's Hearings System in Scotland.

Welsh inspiration

Like Scotland, Wales became devolved from the UK Parliament following the establishment of a new National Assembly (the Senedd) in 1999. Unlike Scotland, however, Wales did not have a separate legal system to England prior to devolution, and justice – including youth justice – was not part of Wales's devolution settlement. As a consequence, responsibility for justice policy was retained by the UK government and the funding situation in Wales meant that, for practical purposes, the nature of youth justice policy was always the outcome of negotiation between England and Wales. A central part of the Welsh strategy was that 'young people should be treated as children first and offenders second' (Haines, 2009). Such an approach contains more than an echo of what might be thought of as elements of a 'public health' approach to children's offending. As Mark Drakeford (2009, p 8), later to become First Minister, put it, in this distinctively Welsh version of youth justice, '[w]hen things go wrong in the lives of children and young people, the Welsh focus has been on trying to put right flaws in the systems on which they depend'.

In addition to the Welsh influence on youth justice, another parallel development was taking place in Cardiff. In the late 1990s, an initiative that has come to be known as the 'Cardiff Model' began combining police and hospital emergency department data on serious violence to fill in the significant gaps in knowledge and understanding of violence when viewed solely through police-recorded crime data. Developed by Professor Jonathan Shepherd, the model involves the identification of key violence hotspots and trends at local and hyperlocal levels, which, in turn, acts as a foundation for police officers, health workers, and other professionals, targeting their resources more efficiently and effectively. The essential characteristic of the Cardiff Model is that it is uncompromisingly driven by data – violence prevention interventions occur on the back of rigorous data analysis, and are refined, scaled-up, or discarded depending on their effects (Centers for Disease Control and Prevention, 2017). Robust evaluations have indicated that the model generates statistically significant reductions in violence (Droste et al, 2014; Shepherd et al, 2016; Jabar et al, 2019). As we shall see in Chapter 2, the emphasis on data that sits at the heart of the Cardiff Model is echoed by some recent initiatives associated with the development of the public health approach to violence prevention in England and Wales.

Serious violence shifts up the political and media agenda

While levels of serious violence in Scotland have remained relatively stable since around 2014, certain measures of serious violence began to rise across much of England and Wales around this time, becoming the source of mounting media and political attention. In particular, the number of detected knife and weapons offences by children and young people began to rise sharply, and the overall proportion of offences that involved the possession of a weapon rose from 2015 onwards (Grimshaw and Ford, 2018). Although there was little substantial evidence that violent crime was rising overall, toward the end of the decade there was a significant increase in the number of children and young people convicted for knife-enabled homicide. More generally, police-recorded knife crime rose by over a third (36 per cent) between 2013/14 and 2016/17, and offences involving firearms by 31 per cent, although it was accepted that improvements in police recording procedures accounted for some of the increase (Office for National Statistics, 2023).

These trends, among other factors, led to heightened media and government attention specifically on the issue of violence by and between young people in England generally, and London in particular. From early 2018, journalists and government ministers alike spoke increasingly about the urgency of this issue, and the need for a new, more effective approach to address it. In contrast, there was little political concern about violent crime in Scotland where rates were at a historic low and there was no evidence of an increase in offending among young people (see Fraser et al, 2024). As we will see in the following chapter, this led the UK government to look north of Hadrian's Wall, and to explicitly pronounce its intention to pursue a Scotland-inspired public health approach to violence prevention.

Conclusion

This chapter has traced the long-term origins of the public health approach to violence prevention in Scotland, and the lead-up to its emergence in England and Wales. In Scotland, this approach was grounded in a well-established 'penal-welfarist' tradition, accelerated by a series of youth-focused policy developments in the early 21st century, inspired by US initiatives, and instigated by the innovative work of the Scottish VRU. By 2016, Scotland's public health approach was hailed in the media as a resounding success. Notwithstanding a relatively brief flirtation with punitiveness at the start of the 2000s, Scotland's journey towards a public health approach to violence prevention appears to have been relatively smooth; congruent with long-standing principles in its youth justice system.

Developments over the same period in England and Wales were more complex and took a somewhat different direction. New Labour's 'tough on crime' agenda (1997–2010) involved a heightened focus on 'antisocial behaviour' – particularly among young people – and entailed the introduction of thousands of new criminal offences. Spurred on by their publicly expressed interpretation of the 2011 riots in England, Conservative-led governments then emphasised the role of gangs in promoting disorder and violence, asserting in their rhetoric a particular national problem framed as 'youth violence' – a framing that would remain influential. In among this, and by contrast, youth imprisonment declined considerably, and from 2015 the 'Child First' agenda began to gain traction. It was statistical trends in reported violence during the latter half of the 2010s that re-sharpened policy attention on the issue of violence between young people, and came to be seen as an urgent crisis in need of a new approach. Looking to Scotland, from 2018, regional mayors and the UK government began to use the language of public health. The emergence and development of the public health approach to violence prevention in England and Wales during the years 2018–23 are the subject of the following chapter.

2

Recent developments in England and Wales

The period between 2018 and 2023 saw a flurry of policy developments, which represented the putative implementation of a public health approach to violence prevention in England and Wales. While Chapter 1 looked in broad strokes at longer-term historical developments, this chapter presents a more granular contemporary history that focuses on these crucial six years.

We divide the chapter into four sections. In the first section, we describe how calls for the public health approach gained momentum and influence over the course of 2018, with a consensus forming by the end of the year.

In the second section, we look at how the public health approach was institutionalised between 2019 and 2023, through three key levers: the creation of regional Violence Reduction Units (VRUs) as vessels for the delivery of the public health approach; the establishment of the Youth Endowment Fund (YEF) as a 'what works' centre for youth violence interventions; and the enactment of the Serious Violence Duty, a statutory instrument that compelled local agencies to work together to better understand and address violence.

In the third section, we explore what the public health approach came to mean during this period, and the contention that arose about how it was being implemented. Finally, in the fourth section, we conclude this chapter.

By examining the consequential pronouncements, documents, and decisions made between 2018 and 2023, then, we seek to analyse the form and content of the public health approach as it was developed by the United Kingdom (UK) government, regional leaders, and a range of organisations across England and Wales. In so doing, we lay the ground for Part II of this book, which looks in more detail at the opportunities and challenges experienced by VRUs, as they have sought to bring the public health approach to life in their respective areas.

Through the course of this chapter, we emphasise four related points. First, we establish that there was significant struggle during this period to define what the public health approach is, and should be. Viewed superficially, these six years saw a consensus form around the public health approach, and its ascent into the realms of established orthodoxy in England and Wales. In fact, competing conceptions of the approach were advanced by different policy players for various reasons at different moments.

Second, we suggest that the public health approach was only implemented in a partial and limited form by the UK government during this period, narrowly focused on two predominant components: the enhancement of multi-agency working and the delivery of (typically localised) programmatic interventions. This is in clear contrast to the broad conception of the public health approach we outlined in the Introduction and further expand on in Chapter 5. To use the language of the 'Four Is' framework, the government focused inordinately on interventions and on one aspect of institutional improvement (multi-agency working), while doing relatively little to reduce inequalities or to increase the overall quality and quantity of institutions, services, and social infrastructure in young people's lives. Arguably, young people's interactions and relationships – with their families, communities, and professionals – suffered as a result.

Third, we highlight the prominent role played during this period by more punitive responses to violence, including what could be called 'punitive prevention' –a range of measures introduced that were couched in the language of prevention, but which displayed a degree of punitiveness that arguably contravenes the core principles of the public health approach.

Lastly, building on all three preceding points, we stress the fragility of the public health approach in England and Wales. Differences of interpretation, narrowness of implementation, ongoing tension with competing ideas, and the vicissitudes of politics all leave the approach vulnerable. If the six-year period between 2018 and 2023 laid the foundations for the public health approach in England and Wales, only time will tell how secure those foundations were.

We will return to these four points when concluding the chapter.

From a crescendo of calls to official orthodoxy

In 2018, violence ascended to the very top of the media agenda, while politicians made significant political pronouncements and policy makers produced consequential policy documents. By the end of the year, calls for radically new violence prevention methods came to a crescendo, and a growing consensus formed around the idea of a public health approach.

Troubling statistics, growing concern

Policy developments in violence prevention from 2018 can only be understood in the context of what happened to rates of violence from the early 2000s – and the ways and extent to which these appeared in the media.

Between the mid-2000s and the mid-2010s, violence fell significantly across England and Wales, but received scant political or media attention. Over the period 2003–14, homicides fell 39 per cent (House of Commons Library, 2023), for instance, and hospital data in England showed that assault with a sharp object fell 30 per cent between 2004/05 and 2014/15 (NHS Digital, 2023). Over the same period, homicides in London fell 56 per cent, from 216 to 95 (MPS, 2021). It is not entirely clear why these substantial reductions did not garner more political and media attention, but the 2011 riots in England may well have played a role – the moralised concerns around young people, criminality, and gangs that followed the riots tending to dominate the discourse.

By contrast, the upward trend in violence that occurred between around 2014 and 2018 attracted significant media coverage. The statistics were undoubtedly newsworthy: hospital-recorded assault with a sharp object (often referred to in the media as 'knife crime'), for example, rose from 3,643 in 2014/15 to 5,053 in 2017/18. In

London, homicides rose from 95 in 2014 to 137 in 2018 (MPS, 2021). Particular concern emerged over the increase in homicides committed by young people aged under 24 involving knives or sharp implements: these offences rose 200 per cent, from just 16 in 2013 to 48 in 2017. In December 2017, it was reported that 'knife crime' was at its highest level since 2009 (Drury, 2017).

The early months of 2018 saw a spate of knife-related crime and homicides across London, and several media outlets picked up on the fact that London's homicide rate had (if only temporarily) surpassed that of New York (Brown, 2018). On 5 April, six stabbings in 90 minutes attracted significant media attention at regional and national levels (Molloy, 2018). Under public, political, and media pressure to get the situation under control, the Mayor of London, Sadiq Khan, hosted an emergency City Hall summit on serious violence on 10 April 2018, attended by the Home Secretary, Amber Rudd, and the Metropolitan Police Commissioner, Cressida Dick.

The Serious Violence Strategy (April 2018)

In the same month, the Serious Violence Strategy was published (Home Office, 2018b), representing the government's official response to rising violence. Framed as addressing 'recent increases in knife crime, gun crime and homicide', the strategy was described as a transformational approach to violence, with phrases such as 'major shift' and 'real step-change' appearing in the accompanying press release (2018e).

The strategy promoted concepts and aims that are broadly in line with the public health approach to violence prevention, without referring to it by name. In her introduction, the Home Secretary, Amber Rudd, acknowledged that 'we cannot arrest our way out of' serious violence, and asserted that 'tackling serious violence requires a multiple-strand approach involving police, local authorities, health and education partners to name but a few' (Home Office, 2018b, p 7). The strategy's 'overarching message' was that 'tackling serious violence is not a law enforcement issue alone', and that it 'requires a multiple-strand approach involving a range of partners across different sectors', but the existence of the public health approach – including its previous implementations, such as in Scotland – was not acknowledged (Home Office, 2018b, p 9). The only reference to public health in the document is in relation to police and crime commissioners developing 'strong links' with directors of public health, 'particularly with regards to drug and alcohol treatment and prevention services' (Home Office, 2018b, p 71). There was no discussion of new national or regional structures to deliver the strategy, aside from a 'county lines'[1] coordination centre. The idea of VRUs generally, and the work of the Scottish VRU more specifically, did not feature.

Despite this dearth of direct references to the public health approach, the measures advocated in the strategy gave an indication of the Home Office's core priorities in relation to violence prevention, which would remain prominent once the government announced its adoption of the public health approach the following year. Two components are particularly notable: enhancing multi-agency working and promoting evidence-based interventions. Regarding the former, the Home Office (2018b, p 71) advocated bringing 'health and education partners into closer partnership with the police to ensure we maximise the multi-agency response and approach', foreshadowing the legal duty to collaborate (discussed later in this chapter).

In relation to evidence-based interventions, the strategy document announced an £11 million Early Intervention Youth Fund, which police and crime commissioners and community safety partnerships could bid into, in order to deliver preventative interventions with young people. Significantly, the strategy also stated that 'no UK interventions were identified that had measured effects on serious violence' (Home Office, 2018b, p 41). The word 'measured' is crucial here – the strategy suggested that, by comparison to the United States (US), the UK did not have a track record of quantitatively measuring the outcomes of violence reduction interventions. This call for more quantitative evidence of interventions' efficacy would gain momentum in the following years, as we will see.

Mounting media pressure and calls for change

High rates of violence continued in the following months, even attracting comments from the-then US President, Donald Trump.

Trump took aim at Khan, claiming that a 'once very prestigious' London hospital had 'blood all over the floors', adding that 'they say it's as bad as a military war-zone hospital' (Smith and Grierson, 2018). In June 2018, under further pressure from additional high-profile murders of teenagers involving the use of knives, Khan hosted another summit, this time focused squarely on London and knife crime. The event brought together representatives from a wide range of organisations, including local authorities, the probation service, the Youth Justice Board, NHS England, young people, charities, police officers, and members of the London Assembly. Among other things, the summit provided a clear indication that, from Khan's perspective, violence was a complex problem requiring coordinated action – at the very least, tackling it demanded more than policing and enhanced enforcement alone.

In among the usual media sensationalism, there emerged a stream of prominent voices from mid-2018 calling for a different kind of response to violence – specifically 'name-checking' the public health approach, and often citing the work of the Scottish VRU in particular. In June 2018, the *Guardian* journalist, Gary Younge, published an article entitled 'The radical lessons of a year reporting on knife crime', as the culmination of his 'Beyond the Blade' series. Its conclusion was clear:

> [T]he most effective way to deal with 'knife crime' is to treat it as a public health issue, and to tackle all the contextual elements – housing, employment, mental health, addiction, abuse, as well as crime – that make some people and communities more vulnerable to it. But that would take public spending and a coordinated and compassionate strategy that focuses on it for the long term. (Younge, 2018)

In this passage, then, approaching violence (or 'knife crime' – inverted commas in the original) as a public health issue seems to involve three main components: addressing the wide-ranging 'contextual elements' that heighten the chances of violence; coordination of government activities (which would involve 'public spending'); and approaching the issue in the long term. The article also included a fourth component: reference to

Scotland's public health approach. A central plank of its argument involved citing the Scottish success story, focused mostly on the work of the Scottish VRU.

Less than a month later, on 18 July, the front page of the *Evening Standard* (London's most prominent newspaper) was dedicated to an article by David Cohen (Cohen, 2018), with the headline 'Violent London: Treat crimewave like public health emergency, experts say'. Cohen's piece summarised the key recommendations of the cross-party parliamentary Youth Violence Commission's interim report, published that day (and discussed further later in this chapter) – the centrepiece of which was the recommendation that London should adopt a Scottish-inspired public health approach to violence prevention (Youth Violence Commission, 2018). Later in Cohen's piece, the public health approach is defined as follows:

> The public health model recognises that most people involved in serious youth violence have a history of trauma. It understands that police tactics – from stop and search to stiffer sentences – can be only part of the solution. Instead, it seeks to approach youth violence with the same preventative and wrap-around care you would deploy to contain and disrupt the outbreak of an epidemic, but instead of cholera or HIV, here the 'infectious disease' is violence. (Cohen, 2018)

The broad message of Cohen's article was similar to Younge's: calling for something radically different and asserting the need to address the multifaceted causes of violence. When putting forward a definition of the public health approach, however, their conceptualisations have little in common – Cohen suggested that its central components are recognition of trauma, going beyond policing, and preventative 'wrap-around care'. The primary commonality of their two articles was not their description of what the public health approach entails, but their reference point for its success: Scotland.

The Youth Violence Commission's interim report (July 2018)

Cohen's piece accompanied an interim report produced by the cross-party parliamentary Youth Violence Commission. The

Commission comprised Members of Parliament (MPs) from the Labour, Conservative, Liberal Democrat, and Scottish National parties, and had been set up in 2017 to better understand the problem of violence in young people's lives and how government could best respond to it. The Commission's interim report advocated strongly for a national public health approach, based on the Scottish model.[2]

In the introduction to the Commission's 2018 interim report, its Chair, MP Vicky Foxcroft, expressed support for certain elements of the Ggovernment's Serious Violence Strategy:

> We were particularly pleased to see the Government recognising: the impact on young people of childhood trauma and adverse experiences, the importance of early intervention in preventing violence later in life and the need for greater integration of services (what is often termed the 'public health approach'). (Youth Violence Commission, 2018, p 3)

Foxcroft effectively described the strategy, then, as calling for a public health approach in all but name. Building on this, the first and most prominent recommendation of the Commission's report was 'developing a national "public health model"'. In advocating for this, the report stated that 'Scotland's VRU is widely recognised as the UK's most successful example of a public health approach to violence reduction' (Youth Violence Commission, 2018, p 6).

The report notes the growing ubiquity of reference to the public health approach in debates about violence, but concern about its potential dilution:

> The notion of a 'public health model' as the ultimate solution to violence reduction is now habitually raised in debates and policy discussions. The Commission supports the view that a holistic and integrated system of care is the best way forward and we welcome the fact that several schemes, which include elements of a public health approach, are being trialled across the country. There is, however, an increasing risk that the term 'public health model' is being used without

> a proper understanding of what is actually required to affect [*sic*] lasting change. As we learnt from Scotland's success, a public health approach requires whole-system, cultural and organisational change supported by sustained political backing. Anything short of this will fail. (Youth Violence Commission, 2018, p 6)

For the Commission, then, the key to avoiding failure in the implementation of the public health approach was sustained political commitment and learning from Scotland. These comments were featured on the front page of the *Evening Standard*, in the run-up to a momentous fortnight of political announcements in favour of the public health approach.

The public health approach achieves consensus: 'everyone has signed up'

By early October, London's Mayor, Sadiq Khan, had announced that London would be adopting a public health approach to violence prevention and setting up its own VRU (Mayor of London, 2018). The-then Home Secretary, Sajid Javid, had also announced a consultation 'on a new legal duty to underpin a public health approach' (Home Office, 2019b). Having replaced Amber Rudd as Home Secretary in late April, Javid's tenure coincided with a marked change in the framing of the government's approach to violence: although continuing to pursue the key measures outlined in the Serious Violence Strategy – such as multi-agency working and evidence-based interventions – these were now couched in the language of the public health approach.

On 13 December 2018, the House of Commons held a dedicated debate on the 'Public Health Model to Reduce Youth Violence' (Hansard, 2018), which cemented the public health approach as the newly established orthodoxy in how violence should be addressed. Early in the debate, the Crime Minister, Victoria Atkins, said:

> The Serious Violence Strategy ... sets out the cross-governmental, multi-agency approach to the public health model ... it places a new emphasis on early

intervention and prevention, and it aims to tackle the root causes of the problem, alongside ensuring a robust law enforcement response ... we are supporting a multi-agency public health approach to tackling the issue and investing heavily in tackling the root causes of the problem and consulting on further measures to underpin the public health approach, to ensure that everyone is working collectively to stop this violence. (Hansard, 2018, column 460)

The Serious Violence Strategy was repackaged, then, as an unequivocal commitment to the public health approach, defined by multi-agency working, early intervention and prevention, and tackling root causes.³ Not to be forgotten, however, was the ongoing necessity of 'a robust law enforcement response'.

In the ensuing discussion, there was frequent mention of Scotland and the 'Glasgow model' – aided by the presence of four MPs from Glasgow. And, by the standards of a House of Commons debate, there was a substantial degree of agreement – a point emphasised by Liberal Democrat MP, Sir Ed Davey: 'There is consensus that the old approach of arresting everyone and putting them in prison is not going to work. We have to have a holistic public health approach, and I think that everyone has signed up to that' (Hansard, 2018, column 476).

Thus, 2018 was characterised by increased media coverage of worrying violence trends, high-profile summits, significant policy documents, and a growing number of journalistic and political voices advocating for a public health approach. By the end of the year, a consensus had formed around the wisdom of adopting the public health approach to violence prevention – if not around what precisely this approach should entail.

May and Javid outline their version of the public health approach

In early 2019, the ascent of the public health approach to official government orthodoxy was rubber-stamped in announcements and publications by the Prime Minister and Home Secretary. In March, when announcing a summit on violence at No. 10

Downing Street, the-then Prime Minister, Theresa May, expressed support for the work done by the Scottish VRU through Strathclyde Police and Police Scotland, and suggested that a new UK-wide approach would use lessons from it – specifically name-checking the public health approach:

> There has been excellent work done under what was Strathclyde Police, now Police Scotland, using the public health approach. What that does is ensures that all agencies, not just across government, but in local government and elsewhere, are able to be brought together to deal with this issue. (May, quoted in Gourtsoyannis, 2019)

Less than a month later, writing a joint article in the *Daily Mail* with Home Secretary, Sajid Javid, May again asserted the government's intention to pursue a public health approach, repeating the key message around multi-agency working and mentioning the creation of VRUs:

> We are today launching a consultation into a legal duty that will underpin the multi-agency, public health approach, an approach that builds on work we are already doing to stop crime before it happens. For example, we're putting an extra £100million into law enforcement in the worst-affected areas, getting more police on the frontline and setting up Violence Reduction Units. And our new £200million Youth Endowment Fund will provide long-term investment for programmes that steer young people away from becoming involved in violent crime or reoffending. (May and Javid, 2019)

May and Javid thus outlined how the government's public health approach would be institutionalised: through a new legal duty, through VRUs, and through the YEF. Arguably, two of these three components represent a continuation of the Serious Violence Strategy's key tenets – fostering more effective multi-agency working (the legal duty) and promoting evidence-based interventions (YEF). The introduction of VRUs was more novel, reflecting the extent of influence that the Scottish VRU had achieved by this point.

In the following section, we explore how these three key policy measures took shape. By the early months of 2019, the public health approach to violence prevention had become the government's favoured language. But how would this approach be operationalised?

Institutionalisation of the public health approach: VRUs, YEF, and the Serious Violence Duty

Between 2019 and 2023, rhetoric became reality, as central and local governments undertook to bring the public health approach to life. VRUs were established across England and Wales, YEF was created, and a Bill containing the Serious Violence Duty passed through various legislative stages. These initiatives also generated an array of more specific and localised violence reduction measures. When surveying the predominant themes of this wide-ranging activity, however, the government's overriding focus on multi-agency working and evidence-based interventions is again apparent.

What were VRUs set up to do?

In Part II of this book, we provide a detailed analysis of how VRUs have operated since their introduction, focusing especially on the views and experiences of their directors. Here we provide brief context for that analysis, through an initial description of their form and focus.

The London Violence Reduction Unit

As mentioned earlier, the first VRU in England and Wales was announced by Sadiq Khan, Mayor of London, in October 2018. The official announcement stressed that the London VRU would be a vessel for the public health approach and would be informed by the example of Scotland's success. It was established to focus on multi-agency collaboration and 'what works':

> The new unit will improve co-ordination between the Metropolitan Police, local authorities, youth services, health services, criminal justice agencies and City Hall as part of the new enhanced partnership, backed up by the unit. It will also build on what works and share best practice ... The Mayor and his team have over the last few months been carrying out extensive research to understand the approaches taken in Glasgow, where a long-term public health approach to tackling serious violence was adopted ... the Mayor is seeking to build on and learn from Glasgow's successes. (Mayor of London, 2018)

Given that this was the first VRU in England and Wales, and its strategy was devised by the Mayor of London rather than the Home Office, it is worth summarising how the public health approach was defined in the press release accompanying Khan's announcement. For the London VRU, the public health approach amounted to a key set of principles (Mayor of London, 2018):

- Enforcement is not enough. The press release makes clear that enforcement should play an important part in tackling violence, and outlines how the Mayor has been supporting enforcement activities undertaken by the Metropolitan Police. It states, however, that 'there is agreement from all agencies that enforcement alone cannot solve this problem'.
- Early intervention is key. The press release emphasises the difference that can be made 'by supporting the vulnerable at an early stage and giving young Londoners better life opportunities'.
- Localism. The press release stresses the importance of 'interventions at the local level'.
- Data. The press release says that 'at the heart' of the VRU 'is the aim of better understanding the risk factors in a person's early life that can lead to serious violence by using data from health, criminal justice and other public services'.
- Complex causation and structural drivers. In the press release, Khan states that 'the causes of violent crime are extremely complex, involving deep-seated societal problems

like poverty, social alienation, mental ill-health and a lack of opportunity'.
- The need for a long-term approach. Khan states that 'the work of the Violence Reduction Unit will not deliver results overnight. The causes of violent crime are many years in the making and the solutions will take time.'
- Funding for interventions. Khan references 'my new £45 million Young Londoners Fund, which is providing young people with positive alternatives to crime and to help those caught up in gangs to get into employment and training'.

The public health approach, then, was defined here as a bundle of core ideas and methods. Both within London and across England and Wales, these various ideas and methods achieved different degrees of prominence and influence in the activities of violence reduction agencies, and in the public health approach as it has been promoted by central government.

Regional VRUs across England and Wales

Having been announced by Theresa May and Sajid Javid in April 2019, it was not until August 2019 – under new Prime Minister, Boris Johnson, and new Home Secretary, Priti Patel – that details were provided of the funding and priorities for the 18 VRUs that were to be run by police and crime commissioners across England and Wales (Home Office, 2019e).

The 18 police and crime commissioners 'secured their provisional allocation through successful bids' and were awarded set-up funding for the year 2019–20 totalling £35 million across the 18 regions. The role of the VRUs was described as follows:

> The Violence Reduction Units will bring together different organisations, including the police, local government, health, community leaders and other key partners to tackle violent crime by understanding its root causes. The new units will be responsible for identifying what is driving violent crime in the area and coming up with a co-ordinated response ... Each unit will be tasked with delivering both short- and

long-term strategies to tackle violent crime, involving police, healthcare workers, community leaders and others. (Home Office, 2019e)

Alongside announcing these VRUs, Johnson and Patel stated that 20,000 new police officers would be recruited, and all police forces in England and Wales could begin to use 'enhanced stop and search powers' (Home Office, 2019e). Funding for VRUs was accompanied by 'Surge' (later 'Grip') funding for police forces in the same 'high violence' areas, to enable them to undertake regular visible patrols in streets and neighbourhoods ('hotspot areas'), and to deliver 'problem-oriented policing', which focuses on shifting the underlying drivers of violence in particular micro-locations, for instance, through changes to street infrastructure or licensing conditions in a specific area to reduce opportunities for crime (Home Office, 2023).

In March 2020, the Home Office produced detailed 'interim guidance' for the VRUs (Home Office, 2020b). This encouraged all VRUs to research 'the whole system/public health approach to reducing violence', and to visit other VRUs, name-checking the Scottish VRU specifically. It lays out six principles of 'whole system violence reduction' (Home Office, 2020b), as defined by the World Health Organization (WHO), which are:

- focused on a defined population;
- with and for communities;
- not constrained by organisational or professional boundaries;
- focused on generating long-term as well as short-term solutions;
- based on data and intelligence to identify the burden on the population, including any inequalities;
- rooted in evidence of effectiveness to tackle the problem.

In its final section, the guidance states that 'the impact of the VRU will not only rely on increased multi-agency data and intelligence sharing, greater collaboration, and strategic coordination and leadership. VRUs are also investing in interventions which should make a difference to those affected by violence in the area' (Home Office, 2020b, p 29). It then goes on to highlight that, so far, VRUs were spending between 34 per cent and 90 per cent of their funding on interventions, before, lastly, discussing the role of the Serious Violence Duty and YEF (Home Office, 2020b, pp 29–31). In this final section, then, the two core components of the work that VRUs should be doing on the ground are made clear: supporting multi-agency working, including through the new Duty, and investing in interventions, working closely alongside the YEF evidence base.

A further two VRUs (Cleveland and Humberside) were announced in January 2022, bringing the total number of VRUs within England and Wales to 20. In addition, having been funded on an annual basis between 2019 and 2022, the Home Office confirmed that from 2022/23, funding would be awarded on a three-year basis 'to enable longer-term planning' (Home Office, 2023a).

A research and analysis document produced by the Home Office at the end of 2023 (Home Office, 2023c) provided another indication of how the government was refining the VRUs' purpose. It stated that 'there was a particular policy focus for 2022 and beyond' to develop four main areas of the VRUs' work: 'further strengthen multi-agency working; encourage and support the sustainability of VRUs; improve the quality and granularity of data accessed, and the analysis of this; and develop the evidence for high-impact interventions' (Home Office, 2023c, no page number). Thus, once more, the centrality of data-driven multi-agency working and evidence-based interventions is clear.

The Youth Endowment Fund

As referred to in May and Javid's watershed statement in April 2019, the YEF would be another central plank of the government's public health approach. YEF was to be government-commissioned, but run as an independent entity, chosen via competitive tendering. Tender documents produced by the government in late 2018 laid out the purpose of YEF:

> Delivered over 10 years, the Fund will deliver transformative change by focussing on those most at risk of involvement in youth violence, diverting young people away from becoming serious offenders. The

> YEF will be key in supporting delivery against the ambition of the serious violence strategy, providing funding for early intervention, working with the grain of effective local partnerships, whilst improving the evidence base for what works. Our desired core outcome would be a reduction in proven offending with a particular focus on serious violent offending, in comparison to an appropriate control group. (Home Office, 2018d, p 2)

> [YEF] will encourage a public health approach, looking to provide grants in a way that builds the sustainability of local partnerships … [the Home Office] expects the Fund to deliver truly robust, rigorous evaluations of interventions to ensure that maximum learning is derived from the Government's investment. (Home Office, 2018c, pp 1–3)

YEF was intended as a key vehicle, then, for the proliferation of evidence-based interventions for violence reduction, to be assessed via 'cost benefit analysis' (Home Office, 2018c), complementary to local multi-agency arrangements. References to control groups and 'truly robust, rigorous evaluations' make clear the Home Office's adherence to 'what works' principles, and a hierarchy of evidence, with randomised controlled trials as the gold standard (see, for example, Standring, 2017; Jones and Whitehead, 2018; Esmark, 2020). Through the creation of YEF, the Home Office made clear its commitment to one of the components of the WHO's four-step cyclical model of implementation: the thorough evaluation of programmatic interventions. This could be seen, in part, as a response to the deficit of such evidence production mentioned in the 2018 Serious Violence Strategy, discussed earlier: the Home Office lamented in that document the relative dearth of intervention evaluations in the UK, compared to the US (Home Office, 2018a). YEF could be seen, then, as an attempt by the government to replicate the US focus on designing and scaling rigorously evaluated programmatic interventions as a primary means of reducing violence.

In March 2019, it was announced that YEF would be run by private equity-backed charity, Impetus, in partnership with the Early Intervention Foundation and the Social Investment Business (Home Office, 2019a). In October of the same year, after a competitive bidding process, the first YEF grantees were announced, including two licensed programmes, which were to be 'imported' from the US (YEF, 2019).

Over its first five years of operation, YEF has broadened its work, to include the production of 'systems guidance' to influence the practice of state agencies and third sector organisations beyond the delivery of specific programmatic interventions. In addition, its research has identified the role of 'social and economic injustices' and criminal justice policies in exacerbating the issue of violence between young people (YEF, 2020, p 5).

As we will discuss further in Part II, the Home Office has consistently communicated to VRUs the importance of utilising the evidence produced by YEF – with a strong focus on its 'toolkit', which summarises evidence on programmatic interventions.

The Police, Crime, Sentencing and Courts Act 2022 and the Serious Violence Duty

As discussed earlier, strengthening multi-agency working was a central pillar of the 2018 Serious Violence Strategy, and this was followed up by Javid's commitment to introducing a new legal duty that would compel greater collaboration between the police, local councils, local health bodies, educational institutions, and youth offending services. On 14 July 2019 – ten days before he was replaced as Home Secretary – Javid provided further detail about how this duty would operate, in a press release, which framed it as a 'new public health duty' (Home Office, 2019c). After a period of consultation, the duty was included within the Police, Crime, Sentencing and Courts Bill, which had its first reading in March 2021. By this point, it had been rebranded as the 'Serious Violence Duty'. The public health approach was not mentioned in the House of Commons during its first or second reading.

Gaining royal assent in April 2022, the Police, Crime, Sentencing and Courts Act enshrined the new Serious Violence Duty into law, the scope of which placed responsibilities on the chief officers of police for police areas in England and Wales, probation services, youth offending teams, fire and rescue, and clinical commissioning groups in England, and local health boards in Wales. The duty also extended to local authorities as a whole, including district councils, county councils in England, London borough councils, the Common Council of the City of London, and Welsh county and borough councils.

Although the duty does not specify a 'lead' agency or person to coordinate activity – leaving it instead to 'the specified authorities to come together to decide on the appropriate lead and structure of collaboration for their area' (Home Office, 2023a, no page number) – the Home Office funding allocation to support its delivery is granted to local policing bodies. The purpose of the funding is 'to cover the work required for partners to deliver the Serious Violence Duty', and, more specifically, 'to enable local policing bodies to assist the specified and relevant authorities with delivering the duty' (Home Office, 2023a, no page number).

Home Office (2022a) statutory guidance elaborates on how the Serious Violence Duty fits into the government's wider approach to violence reduction. This is summarised as follows: 'The Duty is a key part of the Government's programme of work to collaborate and plan to prevent and reduce serious violence: taking a multi-agency approach to understand the causes and consequences of serious violence, focusing on prevention and early intervention, and informed by evidence' (Home Office, 2022a, p 7).

Again, then, multi-agency working and evidence-based interventions are the primary reference points for the government's approach to violence. The guidance goes on to explicitly encourage local areas to 'adopt the World Health Organisation's [*sic*] definition of a public health approach' (Home Office, 2022a, p 8). As in the 2020 interim guidance for VRUs, the six key principles of the WHO's definition are outlined, along with a reference to its four-step implementation approach. Within a section on rooting work in evidence of effectiveness, the guidance states that 'duty holders should use resources such as the YEF Toolkit, Early Intervention Foundation Guidebook and the College of Policing, among others, to ensure they are commissioning activities which are known to deliver the greatest impact' (Home Office, 2022a, p 9).

While it also acknowledges the value of 'innovative approaches', and the importance of pursuing 'long term as well as short term solutions', the guidance regarding evidence-based commissioning referred to earlier is one of the more prescriptive elements in the document's definition of how to pursue a public health approach. Given the predominant methodologies of the bodies cited in this guidance, the government is clear in their preference for interventions that have been quantitatively evaluated as discrete, time- and place-bounded programmes.

As in previous documents and announcements, the document's emphasis on prevention is tempered by references to the importance of 'tough law enforcement', and that 'enforcement and criminal justice-based activity is a critical part of a public health approach' (Home Office, 2022a, pp 7–10).

This overview of the Serious Violence Duty, from 2018 to 2023, highlights two key aspects of the government's evolving approach to violence reduction. First, although it retained its presence within more detailed guidance documents, the language of the public health approach seemed to wane in prominence during this time – relegated from a top line that was foregrounded in all announcements, to a background feature of its more detailed documentation. Second, the content of the statutory guidance on the duty demonstrates that, perhaps increasingly during this period, the government's definition of the public health approach was tightly focused on multi-agency working and the commissioning of programmatic interventions.

What did the public health approach come to be?

In this concluding section, we focus on a central question: During this consequential period of 2018 to 2023, what did the public health approach in England and Wales amount to? To much fanfare, Theresa's May's government adopted the public health approach as their policy for violence reduction in 2019 and announced how it would be implemented: through VRUs, YEF, and (what would become) the Serious Violence Duty. Through these policy initiatives, what did the public health approach come to be?

It is worth returning to the three core elements of a public health approach to violence prevention, as outlined in the Introduction to this book:

- Ecology of causes – 'the what': recognising that violence is driven not by any single factor, but by a multitude of factors operating at the societal, community, relational, and individual levels (World Health Organization, no date; see Figure 5 in Chapter 1).
- Stages of prevention – 'the when': ensuring that efforts to prevent violence involve an appropriate balance of work at the primary level (before it occurs), secondary level (immediate responses to violence, such as pre-hospital care and emergency services), and tertiary level (long-term care in the wake of violence, such as rehabilitation and reintegration) (Krug et al, 2002, p 15).
- Model of implementation – 'the how': following the World Health Organization's (no date) four-step model: (i) defining and mapping the problem of violence; (ii) identifying the causes of violence; (iii) designing, implementing, and evaluating interventions to find out what works to prevent violence; and (iv) embedding and scaling up interventions that work.

In addition, we introduced the 'Four Is' framework, suggesting that an effective violence reduction strategy needs to focus on: reducing inequalities; enhancing institutions, services, and social infrastructure; delivering effective interventions; and enriching the interpersonal interactions and relationships in children and young people's lives.

Set against this conceptualisation, we now discuss how the public health approach appears to have been defined and put into practice by the UK government. We focus on three key points: limited focus and impact on the ecology of causes, particularly at the national level; persistent punitiveness; and the fading prominence of public health language by 2022.

Narrowness of focus and the neglect of national-level factors

Arguably, the public health approach to violence prevention as it has developed through central UK government activities has focused largely on *how* questions – government initiatives have predominantly centred on promoting multi-agency working and commissioning programmatic interventions. While the Home Office has directed each VRU and each Serious Violence Duty partnership to undertake a local needs assessment, examining the localised drivers of violence, there has been a relative lack at the central government level to address national-level societal factors, which are known precipitants of violence. Thus, it would appear that while the UK government has mandated regional work to address localised ecologies of causes, not as much attention has been given at a national level to tackling the national drivers of violence.

This is borne out by relevant statistical trends, two of which relate to inequality and child poverty, both of which are significant society-level predictors of violence (World Health Organization, no date). In terms of income, the UK remains among the most unequal societies in the world, with inequality remaining broadly stable since 2002 (Department for Work and Pensions, 2023; Organisation for Economic Co-operation and Development, 2024). Child poverty has remained between 25 and 30 per cent since 2002, rising slightly from 27 per cent in 2012/13 to 29 per cent in 2021/22 (Department for Work and Pensions, 2023). While these figures indicate the proportion of children who are affected by poverty, they lack analytic depth regarding the extent of economic hardship experienced by children and families. The Joseph Rowntree Foundation undertook an extensive analysis of what it called 'deep poverty' in 2023, concluding that '3.8 million people (1 million of them children) [in the UK] experienced destitution, the most severe form of hardship, at some point in 2022 ... the number of people experiencing destitution has worryingly more than doubled between 2017 and 2022' (Joseph Rowntree Foundation, 2023). During the same five-year period that the public health approach to violence prevention developed as official government policy, then, destitution in the UK doubled.

Concerns were raised along these lines as early as 2019. A Home Affairs Committee report that year critiqued the narrowness of the government's putative public health approach to violence prevention. It argued that 'the Home Office's youth intervention projects are far too small scale and fragmented compared to the services that have been lost' – highlighting in particular the substantial cuts to 'local youth services and prevention work' that had occurred since the implementation of fiscal austerity measures from 2010 (Home Affairs Committee, 2019). Highlighting the role of adverse childhood experiences (which include poverty) as key risk factors for violence, it suggested that the government was inadequately attentive to this issue. The report concludes that 'the Government's rhetoric on a "public health" approach to violence is not reflected in the reality on the ground, and that there is a serious mismatch between the Government's diagnosis of the problem and its proposed solutions' (Home Affairs Committee, 2019).

In October 2019, the government produced a summary guidance document for preventing serious violence (Home Office, 2019f). An interesting section of this guidance, entitled 'What we mean by a public health approach to violence', appears to be the piece of official government documentation that most directly addresses this definitional point; it further highlights the narrowness of the government's approach. The guidance suggests that violence is a public health issue because it harms individuals' and communities' health and wellbeing, as well as being 'a drain on health services, the criminal justice system and the wider economy' (Home Office, 2019f, no page number). It also strongly asserts the value of interventions: 'interventions to prevent violence, especially those in early childhood, prevent people developing a propensity for violence'. It mentions the need to address 'root causes' and cites inequality specifically. When describing the *how* of the public health approach – what actions such an approach entails – the document stresses the importance of a 'place-based' approach and multi-agency working. This is not surprising given the Home Office guidance is based on a more substantial resource produced by Public Health England (2019), which explicitly equates the public health approach to a local-level multi-agency response: 'a whole system multi-agency approach to tackling and preventing serious violence at a local level, *often referred to as a 'public health approach'*' (Public Health England, 2019, p 4, emphasis added). While acknowledging the role played by structural causes such as inequality, then, the activities prescribed by the Home Office guidance were limited to addressing the individualised symptoms of these structural factors, through multi-agency service collaboration and programmatic interventions.

In the summer of 2020, the Youth Violence Commission produced its final report, which focused heavily on the fledgling development of VRUs. While welcoming the creation of regional VRUs, the report expressed two key concerns about how they had been set up. First, short-term funding for VRUs and pressure to spend money in haste were 'resulting in short-sighted attempts to achieve immediate (yet inevitably elusive) results' (Youth Violence Commission, 2020, p 61). Second, and closely related, VRUs were often acting 'primarily as commissioning bodies for local-level violence reduction initiatives', rather than working together as a network to 'promote the national level policy changes that are equally crucial in securing lasting reductions in serious violence' (Youth Violence Commission, 2020, p 61). The report's primary recommendations reflect this – including a call for VRUs to have 'funding projections for a minimum of ten years', and for them to have a clear role in promoting 'national level policy changes' to reduce violence (Youth Violence Commission, 2020, p 62).

Viewed in this way, the government's version of the public health approach neglected national-level social conditions that predictably breed violence. Arguably, their activities undertaken in the name of the public health approach amounted to an array of remedial, often short-term measures to address the localised symptoms of national social problems. In addition, the extent to which the government's formal adoption of the public health approach in 2019 resulted in a substantial shift in policy direction is questionable. The establishment of VRUs and YEF and the creation of the Serious Violence Duty were of course all significant developments, but the primary methods advanced by government to reduce violence through these initiatives – enhanced multi-agency working and the promotion of programmatic interventions – were not novel.

In the language of the 'Four Is' – inequalities, institutions, interventions, and interactions – the government focused inordinately on the delivery of interventions and on enhancing inter-institutional working. They did very little to address the 'macro social determinants' of violence (Bellis et al, 2017). On the contrary, successive governments undertook ongoing austerity measures, which sharply reduced the quality and quantity of services and social infrastructure for young people. In so doing, it did not create conducive conditions for the enrichment of consequential interactions and relationships in young people's lives, whether with their families, their communities, or supportive professionals.

Persistent punitiveness?

It is important to note that this chapter has so far focused narrowly on those aspects of policy that the government have announced and delivered with explicit reference to the 'public health approach'. The broad category of government-mandated violence reduction activities, however, extends beyond those initiatives that they have packaged into their public health approach. Since 2018, the government have frequently stressed the importance of 'tough enforcement' measures to reduce violence, emphasising the role that policing tactics can and should play.

In addition, there has been a vein of government policy during this period that has operated adjacent to the government's public health agenda, which could be described as 'punitive prevention'. While still focused on preventing violence – as opposed to just responding to it – these measures have tended to involve intensive, intrusive policing in particular neighbourhoods, and the sharp restriction of liberties for those deemed to be potential perpetrators of violence. Between 2019 and 2022, for instance, there was an 85 per cent increase in police stop-and-search use (Home Office, 2022b), and successive home secretaries have given both rhetorical backing and additional powers for police forces' extensive use of stop and search. In 2022, the-then Home Secretary, Priti Patel, gave the police more discretion in their use of section 60, which enables police to undertake suspicion-less stop and searches within a given period in a specified area. Patel changed the guidance so that section 60 could be authorised when police anticipate that serious violence 'may' occur rather than 'will' occur (Home Office, 2022b). In June 2023, Patel's successor, Suella Braverman, wrote to the chief constables of all 43 police forces in England and Wales, to give her full backing for them to use all stop-and-search powers at their disposal – describing it as a 'common sense policing tactic' (Home Office, 2023a).

In addition, since 2019, the government have introduced two new court orders that allow the police to significantly restrict the liberties of individuals who are deemed to be potential perpetrators of violence: 'Knife Crime Prevention Orders' (KCPOs) and 'Serious Violence Reduction Orders' (SVROs). KCPOs can be imposed on anyone over the age of 12, if, on the balance of probabilities, the person in question is deemed to be in possession of a bladed article in a public place without good reason, on at least two occasions. KCPOs allow for restraints to be placed on suspects, such as limiting their social media activity to prevent gang rivalries escalating online. In addition to limiting social media use, KCPOs allow courts to impose curfews and geographical restrictions on suspects, and prohibit suspects from being with particular people (Home Office, 2021).

SVROs can be imposed on any person aged 18 or over who has been convicted of an offence involving the use of a bladed article or other offensive weapon, or who had such a weapon with them when an offence was committed. They can also be imposed on those convicted of an offence that did not involve the use or possession of a bladed article or other offensive weapon, where it is found on the 'balance of probabilities' that the person knew or ought to have known that another person would use or be in possession of such a weapon in the commission of an offence (Bridges, 2021). This provision, that an individual could be punished when a court decides they probably knew about another person committing a weapon-enabled offence, brings with it all the well-established issues with 'joint enterprise' convictions, and in fact may represent an exacerbation of them, given the looseness with which the phrase 'knew or ought to have known' may be interpreted (Bridges, 2021). Young people subject to SVROs can be stopped and searched at any time and in any place, without the requirement for the police officer to have 'reasonable grounds'. SVROs can last for a minimum of six months and up to a maximum of two years, and be renewed and extended further on the application of the police. Perhaps predictably, both of these orders have been subject to substantial critique (Billingham and Irwin-Rogers, 2021; Bridges, 2021).

Even at the peak of the government's enthusiasm for the public health approach, its description of how it was reducing violence focused more on enforcement than prevention. In June 2019, when Sajid Javid was still Home Secretary, the Home Office produced a 'fact sheet' about its approach to violence reduction (Home Office, 2019b). The fact sheet consisted of 24 bullet points summarising what the government had done to reduce violence, over half of which were focused on policing, sentencing, and legislative changes to ensure that there was a 'tough law enforcement' response (Home Office, 2019b).

A fragile, fading policy paradigm?

The shifting language from a 'public health duty' to a 'Serious Violence Duty' within the Police, Crime, Sentencing and Courts Bill mentioned earlier could be indicative of a wider issue: the fading potency of the public health approach as a policy paradigm – or at least as key policy language – for violence prevention. When further funding was announced for VRUs in April 2022, for instance, the Home Office chose to describe them as vessels for a 'whole-system approach', rather than referencing the public health approach. In a House of Commons debate on 19 June 2023, Labour MP Dawn Butler critiqued the-then Home Secretary Suella Braverman's over-reliance on stop-and-search tactics, saying: '[Scotland] reduced its knife crime by 69 per cent by using a public health approach. Why is the Home Secretary not using a public health approach?' (Hansard, 2023, column 575). Braverman's response, after defending the importance of stop and search, concluded as follows:

> Obviously, we work with all agencies, because stopping crime needs a multidimensional, multi-agency approach. That is what our violence reduction units are all about; that is what our Grip funding is all about; that is what our safer streets funding is all about—bringing together all the relevant agencies to prevent crime in the first place. (Hansard, 2023, column 575)

Braverman, then, chose not to suggest that the government were in fact delivering a public health approach – instead referring to 'a multidimensional, multi-agency approach', and suggesting that this is what VRUs had been tasked to pursue.

Conclusion

Through the course of 2018–23, the public health approach obtained the status of orthodoxy within the UK government's policies on violence prevention. These policies, however, were dominated by a focus on local-level programmatic interventions and multi-agency working, as opposed to representing a comprehensive implementation of a truly holistic public health approach. The latter would have required far greater attentiveness to: the national-level ecology of causes (especially societal inequalities); all stages of prevention (including work to address structural determinants); and the overall quality and quantity of institutions, services, and social infrastructure in children and young people's lives. The macro-social determinants of violence were arguably exacerbated during this period, and ongoing austerity policies sharply restricted public provision for children, young people, and families. By the end of this period, the language of the public health approach appeared to lose weight and credibility within government.

Part II of this book centres on VRUs. Framed by their creators as key vehicles to advance a public health approach to violence prevention – and working within the broader policy context outlined in this chapter – VRUs have attempted to prevent violence in their local areas through various means. As we shall see, while VRUs have made notable strides in recent years, their ability to succeed is being compromised by central government's narrow and limited interpretation of the public health approach, which neglects societal-level drivers of violence.

At the time of writing, with their latest central government funding settlements imminently due to expire, the future of VRUs remains uncertain. In the following chapters, we reflect on the work of these units during their early years of operation, examine the opportunities and challenges they have faced, and explore their potential role and value in advancing a truly holistic public health approach to violence prevention.

PART II
Violence Reduction Units

3

Bedding in, reaching out

In September 2018, the Mayor of London, Sadiq Khan, announced that he was putting an initial £500,000 towards the establishment of a London Violence Reduction Unit (VRU), to 'lead and deliver a long-term public health approach to tackling the causes of violent crime' (Mayor of London, 2018). Within six months, the Home Office followed suit and announced a total of £35 million in grant funding for 18 police and crime commissioners to establish (or, in the case of London, build on existing) regional VRUs. The Home Office used data on hospital admissions for assaults with a knife or sharp object to identify the areas most affected by serious violence, and subsequently distributed funding to the 18 police and crime commissioners in proportion to the perceived scale of the problem (see Table 1). In 2022, the Home Office gave grant funding to an additional two police and crime commissioners to establish VRUs in their regions. At the time of writing, therefore, a total of 20 VRUs are in operation across England and Wales.

Part II of this book traces the development of these 20 VRUs, from their establishment up until September 2023 when the authors of this book organised and hosted a face-to-face, all-day workshop with VRU directors and members of their teams. Its purpose is to provide readers with a detailed insight into the work of the VRUs, including their priorities, ways of working, and key challenges and opportunities. This chapter begins by examining the early weeks and months of the VRUs, considering the initial structure and make-up of these units, as well as some of the early pressures they faced. It proceeds to explore one of their core functions: enhancing multi-agency working in their respective regions. As part of this exploration, we consider the initial impact and longer-term implications of the statutory 'Serious Violence Duty', which came into effect in January 2023. Finally, we examine the work that VRUs have done to reach out to, and engage with, communities and young people in their areas as part of their efforts to prevent violence.

Establishing the Violence Reduction Units

Many VRU directors commented positively on the flexibility the Home Office had given them to decide on the structure and make-up of their units. This allowed directors to shape their teams in a manner that best supported their visions for the future work and priorities of their VRU, while also enabling them to tailor their team's experience and expertise to match local need. It was clear that most had extensive experience of working in the area of violence prevention prior to their current roles, which ranged from policing and probation, to local government, military consultancy and emergency planning (see Table 1).

VRU budgets were determined by levels of serious violence in each respective region, measured by hospital admissions for assaults with a knife or sharp object (Home Office, 2020a). Broadly speaking, VRUs typically started out by adopting one of two organisational structures:

- **Centralised:** VRUs are made up of a core VRU team leading on strategy and operational delivery, supported by a governance board.
- **Hub and spoke:** VRUs are made up of a core VRU team that develops pan-area strategy and oversight of a number of local VRU teams responsible for local-level delivery. Like centralised models, hub-and-spoke models are also supported by a governance board.

There appeared not to be any consistent factors predicting whether a VRU would opt for a centralised or hub-and-spoke

Table 1: VRU director backgrounds and first-year funding

Violence Reduction Unit	Director's background	Initial VRU structure	Initial year's funding allocation (2019)
Avon and Somerset Violence Reduction Unit	Policing (diversion and restorative justice)	Hub and spoke	£1,600,000
Bedfordshire Violence and Exploitation Reduction Unit	Policing (victims' services)	Centralised	£880,000
Cleveland Violence Reduction Unit	Military consultancy and emergency planning	Hybrid	Established in 2022 with £3,500,000
Essex Violence and Vulnerability Unit	OPCC Project Management and Youth Offending Services	Centralised	£1,600,000
Greater Manchester Violence Reduction Unit	Greater Manchester Combined Authority (Local Governance)	Centralised	£3,370,000
Hampshire Violence Reduction Unit	Policing	Hub and spoke	£880,000
Humber Violence Prevention Partnership	OPCC Policy and Partnerships	–	Established in 2022 with £1,853,000
Kent Violence Reduction Unit	Local Government and Policing	Centralised	£1,600,000
Lancashire Violence Reduction Network	Policing	Centralised	£1,600,000
Leicestershire Violence Reduction Unit	Probation	Hub and spoke	£880,000
Mayor of London's Violence Reduction Unit	Local Government	Centralised	£7,000,000
Merseyside Violence Reduction Partnership	Policing	Centralised	£3,370,000
Northumbria Violence Reduction Unit	Community Safety and Local Government	Centralised	£1,600,000
Nottingham Violence Reduction Unit	Policing	Centralised	£880,000

Table 1: VRU director backgrounds and first-year funding (continued)

Violence Reduction Unit	Director's background	Initial VRU structure	Initial year's funding allocation (2019)
South Wales Violence Prevention Unit	Policing	Centralised	£880,000
South Yorkshire Violence Reduction Unit	Probation	Centralised	£1,600,000
Sussex Violence Reduction Partnership	Policing and Community Safety	Hub and spoke	£880,000
Thames Valley Violence Reduction Unit	Policing	Centralised	£1,600,000
West Midlands Violence Reduction Unit	Local Government	Centralised	£3,370,000
West Yorkshire Violence Reduction Unit	Local Government	Hub and spoke	£3,370,000

Note: OPCC = Office of the Police and Crime Commissioner.
Sources: Home Office (2019c, 2020a)

model, but directors' decisions were based on considerations such as:

- their intended focus – if regional strategy was prioritised, directors tended to opt for a centralised model, and if local operations were prioritised, they tended to opt for a hub-and-spoke model;
- the availability of resources – limited resources sometimes meant that directors found it difficult to recruit the requisite number of staff members into potential spokes to make a hub-and-spoke model viable;
- the extent to which existing infrastructure was already operating at regional and local levels.

Generally speaking, many VRUs seemed to be moving towards some form of hybrid model, which is the type of model promoted in the most recent annual evaluation of VRUs (see Home Office, 2023, p 29 for further details). In short, following the hybrid model, VRUs have a central management team, but devolve some funding to local areas through existing structures (for example, community safety partnerships[1]), or have VRU locality leads who commission or deliver work at a local level.

In the first year of operation, the Home Office set out three mandatory requirements for all VRUs. First, VRUs were asked to produce a strategic needs assessment, which had the dual purpose of identifying the drivers of serious violence in their local areas as well as the cohorts of people most affected by violence. Second, VRUs had to produce a response strategy, requiring them to outline their proposed multi-agency response. This needed to include an outline of the VRU's key members and partners, and a description of how the VRU intended to enhance and complement existing local arrangements that were already responding to serious violence. Taken together, the strategic needs assessments and response strategies were intended to provide a firm footing for VRUs to develop their work, and many directors recalled feeling a sense of relief once these had been produced and published. Lastly, VRUs were required to participate in an independent evaluation commissioned by the Home Office. This evaluation had two primary purposes: (i) to investigate the early implementation of the VRUs through a process evaluation; and (ii) to assess the extent to which VRUs could be subject to an impact evaluation in future years. Some of the findings of this evaluation (and subsequent yearly evaluations) will be discussed later in this chapter, as well as the potential influence that these evaluations had on the work and priorities of VRUs.

Pressure to spend money in haste

Coming into post, VRU directors faced the ambitious goal of reducing levels of serious violence between young people in their respective regions. Many directors described this as a daunting task – a reflection of violence being a 'wicked problem', embedded in other wicked problems that are intellectually, politically and practically difficult to solve (Peters, 2017). Making the task still more difficult, many spending decisions had to be taken before the completion of the all-important strategic needs assessment (see earlier in this chapter). As strategic needs assessments required extensive analysis of existing data, as well as the collection of new data, many of the strategic needs assessment documents were often not complete until VRUs were nearing the end of their first year of operation. Because HM Treasury rules meant that any underspend could not roll over into subsequent years, VRUs were under significant pressure to spend much of their budget before they had access to the results and conclusions of their strategic needs assessments.

Reflecting on the early stages of their time in post, one director said the following:

> The biggest challenge, to be frank, was that there was this pot of funding – ours was £[x] back then, which was meant to be an annual funding settlement – but we had to spend it within six months, which is a bit at odds with the public health approach. So, it wasn't a good six months for us, if I'm perfectly honest. We did well to establish our VRU, but we were commissioning interventions in quick time before we really understood what it was that we needed to commission, so it was a bit of a messy time for us locally. (VRU director)

These sentiments were reflected more broadly across the VRU network. Although directors could do little to avoid a situation in which they were having to commission interventions in 'quick time' without a good grasp of the scale or nature of the problem of violence in their respective regions, this state of affairs represented a striking departure from the principles of a public health approach to violence prevention. Reflecting the World Health Organization's (no date) model of implementation, the Home Office (2020, p 9) interim guidance for VRUs states that adherence to core public health principles require responses to violence that are:

- based on data and intelligence
- rooted in evidence of effectiveness to tackle the problem.

While the problem of commissioning interventions in quick time was one that applied squarely to the VRUs' initial (and not subsequent) years of operation, it is worth noting that the same issue arose for the two additional VRUs that were established in 2022. A number of VRU directors suggested that it would be useful for strategic needs assessments to be completed in advance of any further VRUs being established, so that the directors of any new VRUs could hit the ground running.

Building legitimacy and securing trust

A key challenge facing all VRUs in their early development was to build trust and legitimacy among potential partners, including statutory, private and third sector organisations, and local communities more broadly. For numerous reasons, VRU directors found this challenging. Most commonly, directors emphasised that many long-established organisations were suffering from a form of 'new initiative fatigue', caused by a continual series of initiatives that they had seen come and go in recent years and decades. VRUs, therefore, had to work hard to convince potential partners that they were more than just a short-term political gimmick. As one director put it:

> We were treated with a fair amount of public sector wariness as the new kid on the block, and some distrust from the voluntary charity sector and communities. All in different ways [they] were asking: 'Is this another branded exercise, a shiny new vehicle that is there not to do very much but just to present a different message?' So that was the context to our work. (VRU director)

Accompanying this sense of new initiative fatigue, directors were also acutely aware that VRUs were being established during a time of austerity. With resources among public and third sector organisations severely stretched, VRUs had a difficult task in convincing potential partners that they were there to support existing provision, and that it made sense for money to be channelled through VRUs as opposed to it being allocated directly to already struggling services. Speaking about this challenge, one director suggested that, over time, the VRU had managed to convince multiple agencies of the added value it offered:

> [Statutory organisations] literally heard a big announcement, for us it was £[x], not a king's ransom

> by any means, but they heard that, and I think statutory organisations were not initially happy about it. They were like, 'Well, what are you doing, going to do that, you know, social workers are not going to do?' Fast forwards – they are our biggest champions. They sit around the table with us, as they should do. They understand how we complement rather than replace some of the work that they do. (VRU director)

Many directors spoke about the difficulty of communicating their core purpose to potential partners effectively. While directors sought to convey their essential mission of helping to bring about a long-term public health approach to violence prevention, it was clear that in many cases potential statutory partners and voluntary sector organisations instead saw VRUs, at least initially, simply as pots of funding for commissioning interventions.

> The first point was having to get your partners on board and build trust with partners. We were skating into areas that often people would think were either a police issue, or often you think well, community safety partnerships should be looking at this. And I think you've got to very quickly establish that we're here as a resource and we're here to work with partners – we're not here to reinvent the wheel when I sit at the table. But also, we're not here just to hand out money like Willy Wonka [handed out chocolate], and just to give money out to people and say, you know, 'Just get on with it.' It has to be more than that. (VRU director)

> I don't think people actually got that the VRU is a long-term public health approach – we're not a cash cow. (VRU director)

While some potential partner organisations questioned the extent to which VRUs could add value to existing services, others, such as schools, were often reluctant to engage with VRUs because they felt that the goal of violence prevention was beyond their purview or lay outside their core purpose. For example, some

VRU directors reported to us that headteachers feared engagement with VRUs would give an outward indication that their schools had a problem with violence. In addition, many teachers in schools in England and Wales continue to report high levels of stress and burnout, owing in part to them feeling a burden of responsibility to solve all of society's ills (Toropova et al, 2021) – a situation reflected by the ongoing crisis in teacher recruitment and retention (see Jerrim et al, 2021). In this context, many VRUs found it difficult to insert the issue of violence into an already overcrowded list of priorities. Several directors referred to the broader tendency of organisations to turn inwards during times when resources are stretched, reverting to what they regard as the completion of their core functions.

One common way of garnering legitimacy among partners and building levels of trust was for directors to recruit staff with a background and expertise in the organisation with which they were trying to engage. So, for example, one VRU, which had been struggling to establish good working relationships with local schools, recruited an ex-school improvement officer to lead on the educational strand of the VRU's work. The credibility that came with this person's prior experience, and the professional networks that had already been built up as part of previous roles, granted the VRU a degree of legitimacy and trustworthiness that enabled the unit to begin a positive programme of work across a number of schools in the region. While the development of trust and legitimacy were key to VRUs working effectively with schools, many directors pointed out that trust and legitimacy were the cornerstones of effective multi-agency working more broadly.

Multi-agency working

When the Home Office announced its plans to establish VRUs across England and Wales, the desire to enhance multi-agency working was at the forefront of its outward- and inward-facing communications. For example, as part of the official announcement of regional VRUs in June 2019, the-then Home Secretary, Sajid Javid, stated that it is 'vital that all parts of society work together to stop … senseless bloodshed', and that 'violence reduction units will help do this – bringing together police, local government, health professionals, community leaders and other key partners to tackle the root causes of serious violence' (Home Office, 2019i). In December 2022, the Home Office (2022, p 70) reiterated this position, stating that 'a VRU's core function is to lead and coordinate the local response to serious violence in their areas'. And then in 2023, the-then Minister for Policing, Chris Philp, stated that VRUs 'exemplify [the government's] commitment to working collaboratively' (Association of Police and Crime Commissioners, 2023).

Evidence from a wide range of policy areas suggests that so-called 'silo working' – that is, agencies working in isolation from one another – hampers the effectiveness of efforts to tackle complex social problems (Hood et al, 2017). Preventing violence affecting young people is no exception. By working well together, agencies are better placed to produce numerous positive outcomes, including:

- **Comprehensive understanding.** Complex problems such as violence have multiple causes and avenues for prevention and intervention. When different agencies work together effectively, this invites diverse perspectives and expertise, in relation to both the nature of the problem and its potential solutions.
- **Holistic solutions.** Working as a cohesive group of agencies, professionals are better able to address multiple aspects of a problem simultaneously, increasing the likelihood of successful outcomes.
- **Resource pooling.** Depending on the extent to which agencies are technically able and prepared to pool their resources, combined efforts, whether in the form of funding, personnel, or data, are likely to encourage a better response than any single agency acting in isolation from one another.
- **Enhanced coordination.** When agencies actively collaborate, this helps to prevent duplication of efforts, reduces potential gaps in service provision, and creates a more systematic and cohesive response.
- **Early intervention.** Combining the knowledge and expertise of professionals from different agencies encourages the collective identification of early warning signs that can lead to issues being addressed before they escalate.

- **Tailored approaches.** The higher the degree of collaboration between agencies, the more potential there is to tailor preventative efforts to the specific needs of the individuals and communities most affected by serious violence.
- **Knowledge sharing.** By sharing recent and relevant research and evidence, best practice, and lessons learned, agencies can accelerate the speed at which all professionals learn while helping to avoid similar mistakes being repeated across different organisations.
- **Policy alignment.** Agencies that work closely together will be better able to ensure their policies and priorities complement and reinforce one another's, leading to better coherence at a systemic level and a greater likelihood of lasting impact.

For all these reasons, a core feature of a public health approach to violence prevention as identified by the Home Office (2020, p 9) is the need to ensure that violence prevention efforts are not constrained by organisational or professional boundaries. It is important to note that multi-agency working is best conceived not as a binary case of 'doing it or not', but as a continuum ranging from communication, through cooperation, coordination, and coalition, to integration (Davidson, 1976; Horwath and Morrison, 2007). In this context, the key question is not whether multi-agency working is a good or bad thing, but the extent of collaboration that is most desirable and appropriate in the pursuit of certain goals.

VRU directors were well versed in many of the potential benefits of effective multi-agency working, and it invariably featured near the top of directors' list of priorities. One director, for example, warned against the danger of overlooking the importance of partnership working and falling into the trap of acting simply as a commissioner of interventions (another key function of VRUs as stipulated by the Home Office, 2020b, and discussed in Chapter 4): 'Things like making sure we're taking the whole-systems approach and really bringing the partnership into focus. I think it was very key for me that we avoided just becoming another commissioning body, which I think is quite easy for VRUs to fall into.'

Although some directors believed there was a degree of tension between the roles of enhancing multi-agency working and commissioning interventions to reduce violence, others felt the two roles were compatible and mutually beneficial. Those who thought the latter argued that the money accompanying their role as commissioner of interventions increased their credibility in the eyes of other agencies. Moreover, the experience and knowledge gained from commissioning and overseeing the delivery of interventions enabled VRU staff involved in this process to increase their confidence and expertise around violence prevention.

Challenges to enhancing multi-agency working

While enhancing multi-agency working was seen as one of the most important roles for VRUs, it was also seen as one of the most challenging. A problem raised by multiple directors was that many professionals, regardless of their role or organisation, tended to treat one another as competitors rather than sources of support and cooperation. This led to people and organisations making exaggerated claims about the impact or potential impact of their work, and contests about whose way of working was best:

> There is some fragmentation going on, and in all honesty, the problem is big enough to accommodate as many solutions as we can throw at it as possible. But people overclaim, you know, 'Do my thing and it will all be alright' – it won't. 'Do my thing and stop doing your thing' – well, there's no quicker way of falling out with everyone. (Professor and NHS consultant)

There are many reasons why people are prone to adopting competitive frames of mind, while downplaying others' importance and exaggerating their own. For example, professionals habitually conceptualise social problems from perspectives that align with their own organisation's way of seeing them (Hymans, 2008; Richardson, 2023). This means that people come to value certain ways of understanding and doing, resulting in defensiveness when alternative perspectives potentially challenge the status quo. In these situations, erecting walls and avoiding the possibility of changing one's way of working can be a tempting option or default position. This is especially so when services are operating under conditions of austerity, as has been the case for many years now in England and Wales (see Diamond and Vangen, 2017). When resources are stretched, turning inwards and away from time-consuming engagement with other agencies is likely to place less strain on people's workloads in the short term, regardless of the effect this might have on longer-term outcomes.

Competitiveness is just one of the many potential barriers to multi-agency collaboration, which also include (see Fraser and Irwin-Rogers, 2021):

- legal and ethical issues (perceived and real) around intelligence and data sharing;
- competing visions, priorities, and agendas across different organisations;
- different language, terminology, and definitions being used to frame and make sense of problems;
- the desire for one's own organisation (or oneself) to take the credit for positive outcomes;
- high levels of stress and anxiety among staff, which can drive a culture of retreat and distrust.

One significant problem raised across multiple interviews was the difficulty of VRUs recruiting and retaining experienced and competent members of staff when they could only offer short-term temporary contracts during their initial stage of operation: '[The Home Office] say, 'You're going to get VRU money' ... but it was a last-minute rush again. We lost some staff because people couldn't afford to hang about when they were only on temporary contracts' (VRU director).

This was a direct consequence of the single-year funding agreements that VRUs were subject to during the first two years of their operation. Ongoing relations with external organisations were often compromised because they were founded on personal relationships between specific individuals in a VRU and their partner agencies. The concern of many directors was that when these members of staff moved on to different jobs or came to the end of their fixed-term contracts, this would significantly undermine VRUs' capacity to engage in high-quality multi-agency working.

One of our interviewees spoke about a challenge that stemmed from central government's preoccupation with adopting a 'return-on-investment' type lens through which Westminster-based institutions typically made sense of policy decisions:

> [In England there is] a greater focus on return-on-investment type issues, because ultimately, the Treasury element is based in London. I think that slows things down. People want to know what they're going to get from doing these things. Whereas I think the devolved administrations are more, well, you know, 'This is a problem, this looks like a solution, we can afford to do that for the moment, let's go for it'. The problem with return on investment in violence is the return doesn't usually come to the organisation or the department that spend[s] it ... so you have to have a cross-government approach, so they understand that you're going to get returns, but if health spends the money, you're not going to get it back to health, et cetera, but you'll all benefit in the end. Now, good luck at the moment getting a cross-governmental approach, I'd say, without getting too political. (Professor and NHS consultant)

This quote reflects broader issues around interdepartmental cooperation, which are a perennial problem in central government (Rose, 1971). The point is that effective multi-agency working requires buy-in across multiple layers of governance and operational delivery, from those occupying the most senior levels of strategic leadership, to mid-level managers, all the way down to frontline staff. Resistance at any one of these levels can hamper collaborative endeavours.

Key ingredients to enhancing multi-agency working

Despite the challenges associated with multi-agency working, many directors spoke passionately about the role that VRUs could and should play on this issue. They also spoke optimistically about the potential of surmounting many of the barriers outlined earlier.

Directors stressed that building meaningful connections with partners was time and resource intensive. One director recalled an instance in which she had secured a good working relationship with the regional Director of Children's Services by focusing on their commonalities and promoting a shared vision:

> A lot of it is persuading people who have their own agendas to share your vision. The Director of Education, she's the Director of Children's Services, but the sort of Exec Director for [Area Y], who's a formidable woman ... she said that I sought their views on what their priorities were when we set our priorities, knowing that in the main they would be, if not the same, there would be a lot of common ground. And that's how I did it: I established, a bit like those concentric circle things, you know, where you would think, 'What's the commonality here?', and made that our starting point. (VRU director)

It was clear from the interviews that directors who had substantive knowledge of different agencies, and prior connections with others operating at a relatively senior level, had a significant head start and advantage when it came to the task of enhancing multi-agency working:

> I sat on the Executive on behalf of [Area A] Probationary ... I think one of the reasons why they gave me the job was because I already had some credibility and position amongst the partnerships across, you know, not everybody, but I was very comfortable in that terrain, and therefore able to kind of assume my place, and not feel like I've got to kind of earn it, you know? I was quite comfortable with the notion that this was a contribution ... influencing it strategically rather than trying to run operations. (VRU director)

As reflected in this quote, a number of directors spoke about the specific type of influence that VRUs could and should be having on the work of other agencies, as well as the ways in which agencies worked together. A good example of the type of support that some VRUs were providing to partners included the provision of training webinars, which utilised the expertise within VRUs to deliver sessions on subjects such as trauma-informed approaches, the local drivers of serious violence, and best practice in evaluation (see further Home Office, 2023).

Recognising the problems associated with single-year funding – an issue that had been highlighted in the cross-party Youth Violence Commission's final report (Irwin-Rogers et al, 2020) – the Home Office pushed hard with the Treasury to secure multi-year funding agreements for VRUs. In April 2021, it was officially announced that VRUs would receive three-year funding agreements. Many directors stressed that three-year funding agreements were still far from ideal in the context of their attempts to develop long-term public health approaches to violence prevention. Nonetheless, these agreements did enable VRUs to move many staff from temporary to permanent contracts. This had the dual benefit of attracting high-quality applications for new posts, and increasing the likelihood of retaining members of staff for longer terms:

> It's grown over time and we're now at a point where I'm really happy to say that everybody has permanent contracts. So, one of the key things that's happened with the Home Office funding last year was a three-year settlement, which was really helpful to establish more sustainable approaches, and obviously, retain skilled staff. (VRU director)

> [The multi-year funding] is a real benefit definitely in respect to the team and the sustainability there, and the relationships that have been built up there to be able to fix them in post for the three years. And in the main it sort of changes everything really, when we're looking at the partnership approach ... I think it gives us a real opportunity to have a look at what we can see is working, where there are those roots of things starting to really embed and go well, and then look at what we can follow forward. (VRU director)

Bolstered by the benefits of multi-year funding, then, many VRU directors reported that their teams had started to make significant progress in enhancing multi-agency working in their respective regions. These self-reports were supported by an inspection by His Majesty's Inspectorate of Constabulary and Fire and Rescue Services, which found that in police force areas without a VRU, organisations tended to share information less efficiently (His Majesty's Inspectorate of Constabulary and Fire and Rescue Services, 2023).

Research on multi-agency working has consistently identified the importance of support from senior leaders across each of the relevant authorities (Atkinson et al, 2002; Sloper, 2004; Solomon, 2019). Whereas initially many VRUs had struggled to secure collaboration at a high level of seniority, they were increasingly finding that 'chief execs' and 'senior people' were willing to set aside their time to plan, strategise, and collaborate around violence prevention:

> What we need to have are venues where people can actually feel that they're working together, and then when they leave, they're still working together ... it's an ongoing battle. So, you know, we want chief execs at the strategy level ... we are getting more senior people there than we did once upon a time. (VRU director)

The importance of leadership

All VRU directors agreed that improving violence prevention strategies required not only multiple agencies working together, but effective leadership. From across all of our interviews, we identified three primary dimensions of effective leadership. The first is what we call *system leadership*. This involves a credible lead organisation establishing a clear vision that can be shared across sectors, enabling a sense of unified purpose despite institutional barriers. The second is what we have termed *relational influence*, involving the formation of a 'coalition of the willing' between individuals working across different organisations. As one former VRU director put it: 'Unless you've got people behind you or beside you, you're just someone out for a walk, you know, in leadership. So you must bring people with you' (former VRU director). Third, directors identified the role of *individual personalities* in shaping both relationships and systems. As one director summarised:

> My view in terms of system change and partnership work in general at that level is that it takes time; it takes personalities sometimes to get those big wins. And we are certainly making strides through our board and our partnership in doing some of the same things that others are achieving, who have got a committed director. (VRU director)

In discussions of systems leadership, relational influence, and individual personalities, a frequent reference point in interviews was the example set by the Scottish VRU. In terms of *system leadership*, the Scottish approach has been characterised as a 'whole-system, cultural and organisational change' (Youth Violence Commission, 2018) that instigated a 'growing chorus' of voices who began to speak in the language of trauma and prevention (Fraser and Gillon, 2023; Fraser et al, 2024). This was facilitated by political support from successive Scottish government administrations. In the context of *relational influence*, the Scottish VRU was able to connect with policy makers and practitioners alike, using story-telling, oratory, and publicity to change the conversation on violence – this mirrored a shift in Scottish political rhetoric towards a more compassionate era of justice (McAra and McVie, 2013). Crucially, participants pointed to the significance of *individual personalities* in establishing this form of leadership. The previous directors of the Scottish VRU, John Carnochan and Karyn McCluskey, were often described by interviewees as 'charismatic'. As one participant put it: 'I think it mattered that John was a six-foot Glasgow cop, and he felt cop-ish. And it mattered that Karyn was a woman and that she was bolshie [rebellious]' (academic and researcher).

In a similar vein, 'generous leadership' has been identified as a key ingredient in multi-agency working (see Big Lottery Fund, 2018, p 5; Fraser and Irwin-Rogers, 2021, p 15). Such leadership often involves openness, curiosity, and vision, alongside flexibility, commitment, and trust.

When rooted in accountable and credible organisations, data from the 'Public Health, Youth and Violence Reduction' (PHYVR) project suggest that individual personalities can exert a catalysing effect on efforts to build a movement for change. For one director, the role of the VRU was as 'a sort of leadership organisation, to lead a wider partnership endeavour, even that as a model of work was seen as helpful, and something to borrow with pride'. Another noted that their role was to be experimental and 'explorative, innovative to identify areas for system change', but experienced constraints in the form of evaluation and reporting. This director continued that the answer to this conundrum was to be unafraid of being different and speaking outside the conventional wisdom: 'How do you be that system-change organisation, when you're pushing against organisations that really don't want to change, and are working to different budgetary patterns, planning cycles, and masters who all have different requirements for data? ... Just be a pain in their side and agitate' (VRU director).

Other directors pointed out the need to guard against the possibility that a VRU's existence might crowd out efforts from other organisations. In short, the concern was that having a unit dedicated specifically to violence prevention might mean others were inclined to see the problem of violence as already being covered, and something that could therefore be crossed off their list of priorities. As one director put it: 'I think the biggest challenge really is to make sure that violence prevention is seen as everyone's business, and not just the work of a small unit or commissioned service – that genuinely it's something that is cross-cutting across all, certainly public service, organisations' (VRU director).

In the early years following the VRUs' establishment, this proved to be a difficult challenge. Many directors lamented their lack of 'teeth' in terms of ensuring violence was seen as 'everyone's business', instead having to rely on soft power to encourage and persuade potential partners. Aware of this situation, in 2019, the Home Office began consulting on a new legal duty to support multi-agency action. The Home Office (2019a, p 3) went on to argue that 'the proposed duty will complement and assist the Violence Reduction Units in their aim of preventing and tackling serious violence, by providing a strategic platform with the right regulatory conditions to support successful delivery of this multi-agency approach'. The duty has come to be known as the 'Serious Violence Duty'.

The Serious Violence Duty

The Serious Violence Duty (the Duty) came into force in January 2023, underpinned by provisions in Part 2, Chapter 1 of the Police, Crime, Sentencing and Courts Act 2022. The Act mandated that the following 'specified authorities' must comply with the Duty: police, justice, fire and rescue, health and local authorities. The Duty required specified authorities to collaborate and plan to prevent and reduce serious violence, which included:

- identifying the kinds of serious violence that occur in their area;
- identifying the causes of serious violence in their area;
- preparing and implementing a strategy for exercising their functions to prevent and reduce serious violence in their area.

Although VRUs were not mentioned in the Act itself, they were explicitly referred to in the statutory guidance that supported the implementation of the Duty (see Home Office, 2022). The guidance frames VRUs as potential 'systems leaders', stating that 'some localities may choose to use VRUs to lead on the work', while showcasing examples of current VRU-led collaboration.

The vast majority of VRU directors welcomed the Duty in principle, arguing that its legislative bite would help to ensure specified authorities took seriously the task of collaborating and planning to prevent serious violence. In the lead-up to the Duty coming into effect, some directors raised concerns about the perceived lack of clear and sufficient communication around what the Duty would entail, and how it was supposed to be implemented:

> It's a bone of contention for me, the Serious Violence Duty, because the guidance was really poor in my

> opinion. They make reference to lots of Violence Reduction Units and the role that the VRUs should play in pulling this together, but there is no statutory duty placed on VRUs because not every [area] has one. It's unclear for me the role that actually the VRU takes. There's not the money, availability, power I think of a VRU to pull together those agencies to make sure they're complying with the Duty. So, I agree in principle with what the Duty is saying – I think the VRUs are probably already doing it to a certain extent – but the guidance is unclear. I know further guidance is coming out next month, which hopefully should clarify some issues. (VRU director)

Another issue raised in addition to a perceived lack of guidance in advance of the Duty coming into effect concerned the resources provided by the Home Office to support the Duty's implementation. More specifically, some directors felt that the level of resources being provided to support the implementation of the Duty were inadequate, while others felt that they were being directed to spend money on things that were not directly relevant to the task in hand:

> If I were to go to the micro on it, so Home Office, you're maybe aware of the grant funding around the Serious Violence Duty implementation, but they've done another Home Office special, where you've got eight weeks to spend £[x] on interventions to support vulnerable children and young people ... actually how's that supporting the implementation of the Duty? Should we not be focusing more on getting the infrastructure in place, data sharing, all that side of things? (VRU director)

The phrase 'Home Office special' in this quote reflected a perception among some directors that the Home Office was prone to imposing new and often burdensome requirements without providing the requisite time, resources, or guidance needed to fulfil them. Other directors, however, were less critical of the Duty and its implementation, arguing that it offered an opportunity for VRUs to place themselves centre-stage:

> We've been planning for it [the Serious Violence Duty] for a while because I knew it was coming. So, we've actually put it to our board recently. We've got pretty much agreement that we will essentially help coordinate that duty for the specified authorities … they will actually use our existing structures to make sure that Duty comes into effect. So, I actually think that this is a bit of a pat-a-cake for all VRUs really, because it should be very easy for VRU areas to just get this Duty up and running. (VRU director)

Because VRUs were not named as a specified authority in the Police, Crime, Sentencing and Courts Act 2022, there were no guarantees that these authorities would agree to VRUs playing a central role in the Duty. It is to VRUs' credit, therefore, that the vast majority appeared to have been successful in taking the lead on the implementation of the Duty in their respective regions – a reflection of the legitimacy and credibility they had built during their early years of operation.

It is worth noting that some directors feared that the introduction of the Duty might spell the end of VRUs altogether. Their line of reasoning was that VRUs were integral in enhancing multi-agency working in the absence of any formal framework that mandated collaboration. With the advent of the Police, Crime, Sentencing and Courts Act and the Duty, relevant authorities would now in effect be forced to undertake such collaboration, potentially negating the need for VRUs. A number of directors communicated these concerns during our interviews:

> If you introduce a Serious Violence Duty across the whole country, across the 43 forces [in England and Wales], you've developed a structure that doesn't need VRUs because you've set up the strategic links, relationships, and therefore the need for a unique and separately funded VRU reduces. So I think that's an issue and I wouldn't necessarily say that's a wrong

> thing to do because I don't think VRUs were set up to be there forever ... I just wonder whether the Serious Violence Duty is the exit strategy, whether anybody's actually said that out loud, I don't know. (VRU director)

> I've got agreement from the relevant authorities in [Area A] that the way we approach the Serious Violence Duty will be to use the existing VRU structures. And the fact that they've agreed to that I think is good because it could have been an opportunity for people, if they were discontent, to kind of want to build something else. (VRU director)

While in theory there was potential for relevant authorities in many areas to bypass VRUs in the implementation of the Duty, in practice, this had not occurred. Instead, specified authorities in the Police, Crime, Sentencing and Courts Act had invariably utilised VRU-led structures in the pursuit of compliance with the Duty. One VRU director reflected on the positive impact of the Duty in their region:

> I chair the Serious Violence Duty implementation group in [Area A], but one of the things that I will constantly say is the VRU is not a specified authority, it's you, it's down to you. And I think it's really woken them up to the fact that actually they've got this statutory responsibility around the prevention of serious violence. Whereas before there was probably a tendency to turn up to a meeting and go, oh, it's fine, because PCC [the Police and Crime Commissioner] and the VRU team are doing all of this. (VRU director)

The Home Office's desire to enhance the degree of data sharing across different authorities was perceived by directors to be one of the key drivers of the Duty:

> I think what you can kind of read behind the Duty, and the draft guidance that sits behind it, is that the

> main trigger for [the Duty] is this piece around data sharing. And utilising that to I suppose identify, or even if you like want to say predict, risk as early as possible. That's how I read the sort of main rationale behind it and it's very much focused around data sharing. (VRU director)

Prior to the Duty's implementation, many authorities outwardly resisted VRU data-sharing requests on the grounds of ethical and legal concerns. While directors thought there was some substance to these concerns, they suggested that an underlying sense of embarrassment about an organisation's quality of data was often the main reason behind reluctance to share data. One interviewee put it as follows:

> We don't have an admission that one of the greatest fears people have is if they share data we'll all know how bad people's data actually is, but no one can say that because then the secret is out and they may as well have shared it ... they haven't got very good data, it's not been recorded particularly well, and actually someone needs to be honest and say, 'Well, look, let's start sharing data', and just be frank about the fact that that is the process that will improve data quality. (Professor and NHS consultant)

Having sufficient and high-quality data is increasingly seen as an essential foundation of high-performing public and private organisations alike. In a speech by the Chief Executive of the Civil Service, Manzoni (2017) argued that 'data is at the heart of 21st century government ... we've always held enormous quantities of data – now we need to make sure we use it properly'. While there was a clear recognition of the importance of data and data sharing among directors, there was a clear sense that the data collected by VRUs, or to which VRUs had access, were not as robust or comprehensive as directors would have liked them to be. In this context, the Duty provided a useful nudge in helping authorities, including VRUs, push past any lingering discomfort about sharing data.

In addition to helping ensure that specified authorities collaborate and share data, some directors also pointed out that the Duty had prompted enhanced engagement and collaboration from additional partners, such as schools. Although schools were not included as specified authorities in the Police, Crime, Sentencing and Courts Act, specified authorities can nevertheless make 'requests' of schools in line with the preparation and delivery of their violence prevention strategies. Subsequently, schools 'must comply' with these requests, subject to certain provisos.[2] Some directors were pleased to report that many schools were now being compelled to share data, which was particularly useful for better understanding the nature and scale of pupil exclusions, as well as how authorities can best provide support to excluded children, or children at risk of exclusion.

One of the major benefits that directors reported after just a few months of the Duty's implementation was the extent to which connections were being made between issues that had previously been treated as relatively discrete:

> I think what [the Duty] has actually done is pushed that idea of joining up workstreams, understanding that systems change has to happen in order to implement some of what we're trying to deliver long term – that's started. I think we're seeing join-up of exploitation and serious violence and 'county lines' and things like that. There's a sort of movement to understand that these are not separate things, that they are all part of the same conversation. (VRU director)

While the Duty appeared to be achieving its core goal of enhancing collaboration and data sharing across public sector agencies, VRU directors were keen to stress that engaging with and listening to local communities and young people were also a core part of their mission, and integral to achieving significant and lasting reductions in serious violence.

Engaging with communities and young people

In the official announcement of funding for VRUs, the-then Home Secretary, Sajid Javid, spoke about the importance of engaging community leaders in efforts to prevent violence (Home Office, 2019i). Shortly thereafter, Home Office (2020, p 12) interim guidance for VRUs stressed the importance of VRUs working 'with and for communities'. The guidance went on to state that 'genuine community involvement in the VRU – as opposed to traditional engagement or consultation – is one of the things which makes a VRU have the kind of local impact which existing multi-agency structures don't always have' (Home Office, 2020b, p 12).

There are many practical and ethical reasons for paying careful attention to the voices of those living in communities with high rates of serious violence. First and foremost, the nature and impact of violence cannot be fully understood without hearing from those who are affected by it. Foregrounding the voices of young people can help to guard against overly simplistic explanations that sit and remain solely at the level of individual behaviour, neglecting the macro-level structural drivers that underpin micro-level actions (Jones et al, 2021). For example, in a recent project that explored young people's views of violence in five major cities across the United Kingdom, participants spoke at length about the role of poverty, inequality, housing conditions, and unemployment (Hope Collective, 2022a). Taking into account young people's perceptions of the causes of violence can also help to inform appropriate and effective responses designed to prevent it (Chonody et al, 2013; Irwin-Rogers et al, 2020; Dawson et al, 2023). For these reasons and many others, VRUs had typically expended a significant proportion of time and resources fostering strong relationships with local communities and young people in their respective regions.

Many directors echoed the sentiments expressed in the Home Office (2020) interim guidance for VRUs, talking about the need to go beyond a tick-box type exercise:

> I call it the saviour complex – where you think you know what's best for the kids ... I've got lots of people talking about what's best for these troubled kids, these hard-to-reach young people, who are not listening to them, or what's best for the community and listening to them. And I know that sounds, you know, simplistic

but actually I think it's just a systemic thing where people believe that they know best and they wheel people out to give the voice ... in a performative nature, tick a box, and never really listen to what they're saying. (VRU director)

To move beyond something performative, many directors stressed the importance of active participation and co-design, as well as varied and creative methods of engagement, listening, and dialogue:

> Engaging with communities, yes absolutely, and I think going further than engaging and listening to, but actually making sure they're active participants. We've got a few different mechanisms for that. We certainly do an awful lot of qualitative research, and it tends to be thematic. We also have community ambassadors in the VRU, some of them are young people, some of them are older members of the community, who have a real voice around this agenda and can be our sounding board. We've recently introduced a Citizens' Advisory Panel as well, so we've got community as really part of the governance process. We've tried to make sure that that's a strong theme throughout everything that we do. (VRU director)

> In terms of the community-led approach, it's about listening to the community, as it says on the tin, in terms of finding out what the strengths of that community are, what the challenges are, and why those challenges exist in that community. What we want to do is co-design what the funding should be spent on and what interventions that community needs, based on what they perceive is a challenge for them. It's about going in and finding out the strengths and the challenges that exist in each community, doing a number of months of community engagement, doing that a number of ways in terms of parent engagement workshops, youth engagement, walks and talks with

> local residents, and facility to co-design sessions. (VRU team member)

As is reflected in these extracts, directors were keen to highlight the importance of avoiding a working style of 'doing to' and moving instead towards a position where they were 'working with' communities. A shift in the direction of participatory approaches that involve policy makers and professionals engaging closely with communities and young people in decision making has taken place across a broad range of policy areas in recent years, including healthcare (Hurtubise, 2023), local government spending (Pardo-Beneyto and Abellan-Lopez, 2023), education (Luguetti et al, 2024), music and the arts (Stehlik et al, 2020), and the design of public space (Loebach et al, 2020). The rationale underpinning each of these shifts is that close engagement with stakeholders affected by decisions creates a more ethical way of exercising authority and ultimately better outcomes.

Many VRUs had identified and implemented creative and effective methods of engagement, including but not limited to workshops, youth boards, co-designed surveys, and 'walks and talks' in local areas. It was no surprise, therefore, to see directors reflecting on their units' engagement with local communities and young people with confidence and pride.

Conclusion

This chapter has explored the establishment of VRUs and the early challenges they faced. We saw that VRU directors appreciated the flexibility afforded to them by the Home Office, which allowed them to recruit and structure their teams according to local context. However, a significant challenge to all directors was the pressure to allocate funds before fully understanding the local violence landscape in their respective areas. This created tension between the perceived need for immediate action capable of achieving results in the short term, and a more evidence-informed long-term strategy that characterises a holistic public health approach to violence prevention.

In their early months and years, VRUs sought to build legitimacy and trust with local communities and partner agencies.

Directors found themselves having to overcome 'initiative fatigue' among potential partners, especially in the context of austerity where resources were already stretched. In addition, VRUs faced the complex challenge of collaborating with organisations across various sectors, each with its own priorities and competing ways of seeing and doing. Despite this, the multi-agency approach was clearly seen by all directors as a critical strand of their VRU's work. Although a difficult task, it was one that all VRUs seemed to have risen to with a high degree of success.

Another essential aspect of VRUs' early work was engaging with local communities and young people. By prioritising community involvement through various creative methods, VRUs worked hard to ensure that their violence prevention efforts aligned with the experiences and views of those most affected. This was an important part of further building trust and confidence in VRUs and ensuring their work was appropriately tailored to local need.

As we move on to Chapter 4, our focus shifts to another two important functions of VRUs: commissioning programmatic interventions to reduce violence, and working to influence various national and institutional policies that make up the broader landscape of violence prevention in England and Wales. Both of these additional functions are integral to ensuring VRUs fulfil their potential in bringing about a truly holistic public health approach to violence prevention.

4

Aiming upstream, slipping downstream

Having now explored the efforts of Violence Reduction Units (VRUs) to enhance multi-agency working and reach out to their local communities, this chapter considers two additional VRU functions. First, we explore VRUs' role in commissioning interventions to prevent and reduce violence. In short, VRUs spend a sizeable proportion of their budget each year funding a range of interventions designed to reduce violence. Despite many VRU directors expressing a desire to 'get upstream' of the problem of violence − in other words, to focus their attention on prevention and root causes − in practice, they often found themselves slipping downstream into a more reactive mode of working, as a range of factors, including political pressure and the influence of evaluations, drew them away from upstream work.

In the second part of the chapter, we turn our attention to VRUs' role in shaping national and institutional priorities, policies, and practices, which have the potential to prevent violence in England and Wales. This work at the national and institutional level was an important part of the Scottish VRU's public health approach to violence prevention (Fraser and Gillon, 2023). In England and Wales, however, VRUs have encountered significant challenges in making progress in this area. To set the foundations for our concluding chapter, we explore these challenges and consider why VRUs have struggled to replicate the success of their counterpart north of the border.

Commissioning interventions to reduce violence

In its interim guidance for VRUs, the Home Office (2020, p 29, emphasis added) made clear that to prevent violence in their respective regions, VRUs were expected to go beyond the task of enhancing multi-agency working: 'The impact of the VRU will not only rely on increased multi-agency data and intelligence sharing, greater collaboration, and strategic coordination and leadership. VRUs are also *investing in interventions which should make a difference to those affected by violence in the area.*'

The wording here leaves plenty of room for interpretation. First, the phrase 'make a difference to those affected by violence' goes beyond what could have been a more narrowly framed alternative 'reduce and prevent violence'. In other words, the purpose of VRU-funded interventions need not necessarily be focused squarely on reducing violence, but in making some sort of difference. Second, no reference is made to any timeframe concerning the impact of interventions. This is noteworthy, because one of the most difficult challenges raised by directors concerned the tussle between short- and long-term impact: 'There's a real tension between understanding the long-term causes of violence and looking at longer-term strategies to eradicate them, as well as to make sure we are doing something now. That tension has existed since the unit started work and is still very present' (VRU director).

This tension reflects a distinction between what has been termed primary, second and tertiary prevention. In their report for the World Health Organization, Krug et al (2002, p 15) summarised these levels of prevention as follows:

- Primary prevention: approaches that aim to prevent violence before it occurs.
- Secondary prevention: approaches that focus on the more immediate response to violence.
- Tertiary prevention: approaches that focus on long-term care, in the wake of violence.

A distinction was also drawn between approaches to violence prevention depending on their target groups:

- Universal interventions: aimed at groups or the general population without regard to individual risk.
- Selected interventions: approaches aimed at those considered at heightened risk for violence.
- Indicated interventions: approaches aimed at those who have already demonstrated heightened behaviour.

The report acknowledged that most violence prevention efforts take place at the secondary or tertiary levels, and called for greater investment in primary prevention, stating: 'A comprehensive response to violence is one that not only protects and supports victims of violence, but also promotes non-violence, reduces the perpetration of violence, and changes the circumstances and conditions that give rise to violence in the first place' (Krug et al, 2002, pp 15–16). While, in theory, VRUs offer a promising vehicle for driving primary prevention to the fore, directors raised concerns about numerous push and pull factors that prevented this from becoming a reality.

Challenges of prioritising primary prevention

The logic underpinning the drive towards prevention is that if upstream activities can effectively stem the problem at its source, then this will diminish the need for resources to be expended further downstream. As one director put it: 'If we get VRUs right, to be quite honest with you, you wouldn't have to be at the tertiary end ... my idea is that we do more of the early intervention work and the preventative work' (VRU director).

When the Home Office announced funding for VRUs, it outwardly badged the units as a new violence prevention initiative that was designed explicitly to tackle the 'root causes' of violence through 'long term solutions' (Home Office, 2019c). Accompanying this announcement, National Police Chief Council Chair, Martin Hewitt, said 'it is widely agreed that prevention must be the priority' (Home Office, 2019i). This push for prevention was based, at least in part, on events in Scotland, where the Scottish VRU had undertaken a long-term programme of reframing the ways in which violence was understood (Fraser and Gillon, 2023).

A source of frustration and anxiety among directors was the perceived mismatch between the core preventative mission that they had been tasked with on the one hand, and the metrics put in place to evaluate their success on the other. Every year, the Home Office commissions an independent evaluation of VRUs, a key part of which attempts to measure their impact using the following measures:

- reduction in hospital admissions for assaults with a knife or sharp object, and especially among victims aged under 25;
- reduction in knife-enabled serious violence, and especially among victims aged under 25;
- reduction in all non-domestic homicides, and especially among victims aged under 25 involving knives.

While these measures all make sense in the context of much of the VRUs' work, they inevitably fail to capture the potential benefits of certain forms of primary violence prevention – that is, prevention that occurs upstream of the problem and attempts to get at its root causes. For example, a range of early childhood family influences have been shown to play a significant role in the onset of violent behaviour at a later age. These include a lack of adult monitoring and supervision of children, harsh physical punishment and disciplining, and exposure to domestic violence and abuse (David-Ferdon et al, 2016). In addition, growing up in societies with high levels of socioeconomic inequality and child poverty has been closely linked with higher rates of violence later in life (Ludwig et al, 2001; Morenoff et al, 2001; Wilkinson and Pickett, 2009). Given the ages of the children being targeted and supported, the potential effects of VRU interventions aimed at addressing some of these early-life issues could take a decade or more to manifest.

Crucially, many directors expressed feeling disincentivised from commissioning primary prevention work:

> If I'm genuinely going to adopt a public health approach ... you want to intervene early to provide greater protective measures, and alternate pathways in order to enable more positive outcomes. How can

> I achieve that if I have to deliver quarterly statistics against reduction in knife-crime offences, reduction in knife-crime hospital admissions, and reduction in homicides? Because that forces me down the road of tertiary intervention … it becomes more of a mechanism to feed the data-hungry beast of quarterly reports. (VRU director)

> We're not doing true public health, as in, we're not going right back to the early roots because that's too slow … capturing younger siblings coming up … it's a lot slower. So I feel we are playing with the middle ground, and I think that might be where we don't necessarily win. (VRU director)

These sentiments were also reflected in the latest Home Office evaluation of VRUs, which stated that 'there was a widespread view [among VRU staff] that a public health approach to serious violence requires still earlier identification and engagement to ensure it is preventative' (Home Office, 2023, p 51). Many directors argued that establishing a commitment to long-term preventative work was especially challenging during a period of austerity in public services, coupled with the damage done to the economy by the COVID-19 pandemic:

> [Post-COVID], I think there's a massive risk that partners revert back to their own kind of territory and we firefight more and more. The case could never be bigger for prevention, but I think the challenges will be bigger still. There's going to be some intense pressure on services, and I just think it's a bit of a perfect storm really, for us to lose the commitment, if you like, to the public health approach. (VRU director)

The director in this extract equates the public health approach with a long-term preventative strategy. It is worth noting that this sense of being pushed away from preventative activity is reflected in the proportion of VRU interventions falling into the category of primary prevention. In the year ending March 2023, less than a quarter of commissioned interventions were aimed at the primary prevention stage, with the remainder operating at the secondary and tertiary stages (that is, further downstream).[1] The pressure to generate impact in the short term was perceived to be coming both from the Home Office – particularly through the mechanisms of quarterly reporting and annual evaluations – as well as from government ministers themselves: 'When we have had meetings, well it was [government minister] ... he was very clear about, "Right, we met six, eight weeks ago, right, what are you doing about the summer of violence? What have you got in place for right now?"' (VRU director).

> I think there has been a shift since we first started, and probably over the last 12 months, I would say that the Home Office have become far more focused on short-term gains; short-term impact. And that shifts in terms of who are some of the critical partners, shifts in terms of some of the work that we are doing. That short-term impact really elevates the importance of the police, because they are the ones that can have that real short-term impact ... but that detracts from this stated aim of a long-term public health approach. (VRU director)

Another factor that directors thought was pushing VRUs away from primary prevention was the Youth Endowment Fund (YEF) toolkit, which is designed to show 'what works' in violence reduction. The toolkit is based on studies that examine the effectiveness of different types of violence reduction intervention, with research employing randomised controlled trials being held as generating the 'gold standard' of evidence. VRUs are instructed to spend 20 per cent of their grant on what the YEF toolkit describes as 'high impact' interventions, with the Home Office (2023) indicating that this percentage is set to rise in the coming years. Some directors were concerned that they were being pushed too quickly and too strongly in the direction of the YEF toolkit, and that this had the potential to overly restrict VRUs and hamper innovation:

> Sorry, this is a triggering moment for me. Certainly the funding we have got for the next three years

> clearly [sets out that] 20 per cent of funding needs to be on these defined interventions. And you think, okay, focused deterrence, you think A&E [Accident & Emergency] [hospital-based interventions], as examples – they're very much responding after the fact. And again, I'm not saying they're bad interventions, far from it. But all of a sudden, we are restricted, or focused in various ways ... it's almost like, well, why are we doing stuff if the evidence is already there? Is testing that innovative approach not part of what we're meant to be doing? (VRU director)

> We very much see VRUs as having a role in kind of generating more evidence ... I'm sure you're aware of this, the Home Office this year have basically said that a percentage of funding has to be on high impact ... I'm not totally against it, I just think that it was too kind of linear, and too eggs in one basket, and actually too soon, really, to be doing that. So, you know, quite a few VRU areas had to abandon certain interventions in favour of others. And I just think that's a real shame, and I don't think that is consistent with the public health approach – it's as much about generating evidence as it is about using it. (VRU director)

Some interviewees thought there was a balance to be struck between commissioning the evidence-based interventions identified by the YEF toolkit and experimenting with new and innovative forms of work. One interviewee stressed that a 'proper public health approach' meant avoiding a situation whereby one became overly reliant on past data:

> If we keep going back to what's already been done, what's already in umbrella reviews, we're just ... you know, I know it's an overused phrase, but we're very rear-view mirror ... get a narrative, okay, establish the evidence you've got which is strong but you've got to leave enough wriggle room in there for the sort of evidence we need if we're going to get a proper

public health approach in as well. (Professor and NHS consultant)

The Home Office annual evaluations were seen by directors as another major factor pushing them away from primary prevention, as well as more novel and innovative interventions:

> Because of the way that funding comes, and evaluations, we feel constrained to improve on what works, or to continue to deliver what works, but more of it. Whereas, you know, when the VRUs initially started, my vision when we came in was to try new things, understand whether they worked or not, and accept that some of them might not work. Whereas I think the evaluation process has driven us towards the continuance [of] maybe more of what's already there. (VRU director)

> It definitely looked more free reign before and more innovative before, and now it does seem quite prescriptive, and it's almost, just allocating the budget to what's already been set, which I think is a shame, personally ... it feels like they [the Home Office] just want to back winners. (VRU director)

It is worth noting that the latest Home Office evaluation (2023, p 35) does indeed seem to nudge VRUs away from the kind of universal preventative activity referred to in Krug and colleagues' (2002) World Health Organization report, stating that: 'The VRUs' and partners' response to violence should reflect the needs of and target those identified as at risk.'

In addition to the pressure coming from the Home Office, the YEF, and central government ministers, some directors also perceived there to be significant public pressure to bring about short-term results:

> The expectation on us was to spend some money and to be able to evidence what we were doing. I think it is often assumed that was a political pressure, a

> political demand. In fact, it was as much of a public demand. We had been set up in response to the rise in homicides involving young people and a real public fear that our young people were caught up in high levels of violence and were not safe ... and so people wanted to see investment and action. (VRU director)

> To go back to the first six months of the unit, it was simple to me that if we disappeared to develop a long-term strategy with a theory of change, five-year plan et cetera, we would have had lost our credibility and squandered that moment of possibility, of change. There was a public desire to do something now. (VRU director)

While many directors recognised legitimate public concerns for action to be taken in the here and now, others stressed the importance of not losing sight of VRUs' long-term scope and mission. In this regard, one director highlighted the potential role of those they termed 'enablers' in helping VRUs to resist pressure to collapse into narrow, short-term thinking:

> I very much see that as my role, to kind of fight that battle in a really professional way, to use negotiating and influencing skills with people to say, we should not and cannot be reactive. And when you look, especially in [Area A], the [X] murders that we had within [X] days ... there then comes a lot of pressure of, well, 'What are you doing about it?' ... And I think that's my place to have those conversations with my enablers, and I'd say the Chief Constable, the PCC [Police and Crime Commissioner]. Certainly people within the CSPs [community safety partnerships] are in support of me and my [long-term] message, so I've got really good enablers. (VRU director)

Directors, then, benefited in various ways from having key stakeholders around them who were both aware of and bought into the long-term mission of VRUs and the holistic public health approach to violence prevention that they were trying to advance.

Even if directors were inclined to resist public and political pressure, some interviewees highlighted that the potential provision of interventions in the space of primary prevention was lacking in quantity and quality relative to those operating further downstream:

> I think, almost like, the commissioning landscape is not ready yet. So, I've heard on the grapevine about struggles to commission primary prevention, because there's just not that vibrant, sort of, voluntary sector and other landscape of people who are actually delivering this ... it's much better for secondary or tertiary, but early intervention or diversion ... it's probably still not as good as it could be, particularly in terms of evidence-based interventions. (VRU team member)

One senior civil servant, keen to view things through a more pragmatic lens, stressed the reality of VRUs needing to survive in a volatile political environment – a sentiment echoed by some directors:

> The evaluation that was published that said the presence of VRUs has prevented X many violent offences, and this has saved this amount of money – that's big. You don't really have that with most government initiatives. That's really important, because if you can point to something that proves that this has reduced violence, unlike a million other things, I would not get rid of that if I was a minister ... when you are having arguments with the Treasury about what your spending review settlement looks like, they don't want to hear, 'It's just the right thing to do.' They want to hear, 'It's going to save this much money.' So VRUs have a huge advantage there, and that's why I think it's not unreasonable for them to have felt the pressure that they have felt. (Senior civil servant)

> You've got to justify your worth, haven't you? So, if there are things that you know will give you a quick

bang for your buck, then you're always going to go down that route than try to be a bit bolder and braver, and actually look at some of these other areas where it might take a bit of time. (VRU director)

In short, then, although VRUs were explicitly badged as units designed to tackle the root causes of violence – and all VRU directors had ambitions of aiming their efforts upstream – the perceived pressures coming from government ministers, Home Office evaluations, the general public, and the availability of high-quality primary interventions, meant the work of VRUs ended up slipping further downstream. While many felt frustrated with this situation, others stressed the potential political advantages of being able to show tangible results in the short term.

Scaling up interventions

When directors were asked about their future aspirations, most spoke about the desire to scale up commissioned interventions. One director saw a primary role of VRUs as being to channel money and resources directly into grassroots organisations, which they perceived as having the most potential to make a difference in children and young people's lives. From this director's perspective, the greater the proportion of a VRU's budget that could be directed to grassroots interventions, the better:

> I wanted to always give away 50 per cent of what we were doing. I realise now that was a bit of a Jesus complex there because the first year, I gave away 50 per cent to the community, and almost couldn't afford staff. Yeah, so rewind, we do give a fair amount of what we're doing out to the community because, let's face it, I'm very much into grassroots, you know, their reach is much better than ours. (VRU director)

After a long period of austerity and shrinking government grants, VRU budgets could very quickly become swallowed up by the high level of demand for funding from grassroots charities. Other directors were keen to scale up interventions that were currently viewed as effective, but operating only at a relatively small scale:

> So, I think the main kind of exciting opportunity for me would be the ability to scale up things that we know work, and that we can provide the evidence base for, and then think, well, because of that, we're actually going to produce, to prevent that much more harm. Whereas at the moment, I think we've got some good standalone examples of initiatives that aren't scaled up, or if we scale them up, it's only tiny, because we've had a little bit of Youth Endowment Fund money, so it's not a systematic approach to prevention, it's some good practice in one particular area. So, that's the exciting bit to me for the future. (VRU director)

Several directors were keen to highlight the economic costs of violence to society, which fell across various institutions including health, policing, and criminal justice. Seen in this context, they argued that the cost of commissioned interventions, while significant, was good value because of the likelihood that any reductions in violence would cover these intervention costs, and more. There was, however, a significant barrier to scaling up interventions, which related to how VRUs were funded. Two problems were apparent. First, VRU money could not be rolled over into subsequent years, which forced directors to spend the entirety of their budget each year, regardless of whether that seemed appropriate and desirable:

> My understanding is there is a lot of red tape around the Treasury and Home Office, as well as around how the funding works, and that's why we're told we can't roll over funding, because it just can't be done with the way the Treasury works. As opposed to, 'We don't believe in the rationale for it' – I think they would agree there's a rationale there, but it's a bit 'computer says no', which is frustrating. (VRU director)

Second, while the VRU multi-year funding settlement marked a significant improvement on the previous year-on-year funding agreements, directors found it puzzling that their budgets were set to decline year on year, when they argued it would have made more sense to start with a smaller budget, which then increased in future years:

> I think also the most money comes in year one, and we lose [£x million] next year ... so unfortunately, it's almost the wrong way round. It would have been much nicer to have the extra money in year two or year three so you could say, 'Right, we start things this year, because it's not a full year, but year two, everything's embedded, scale it up, really hit it hard with people that have a grasp of what they're doing.' (VRU director)

> Certainly the spending is contradictory because one of the values of a three-year settlement would be that you could start something and build it ... but they gave the greatest amount of money in the first year, which actually, all of which had to be spent in the first year. So you create a scaling-down effect. (VRU director)

In short, while VRU directors expressed a clear desire to scale up the best of their commissioned interventions, practical constraints meant that this was likely to be a difficult task in the years ahead.

Evaluations and reporting

Since the early 1980s, public sector institutions across much of continental Europe and anglophone countries have been shaped by principles associated with New Public Management (NPM). Among these principles is a results orientation underpinned by performance metrics and evaluation (see Norris and Kushner, 2007; Esmark, 2020). Many aspects of the relationship between central government and the regional VRUs reflect this, most notably in the form of the ongoing annual evaluations commissioned by the Home Office. Beginning with an initial 'impact evaluation feasibility study' in the first year of VRUs' operation, the Home Office has subsequently sought to evaluate VRUs' work in part based on their success in meeting a number of key performance indicators (KPIs), including the reduction of hospital-based admissions for knife assaults and non-domestic homicides (see Home Office, 2020a). At the same time, through these same reports and the interim guidance provided to VRUs, the Home Office has encouraged VRUs to ensure the interventions they commission are evaluated (Home Office, 2020b).

The potential benefits of infusing evaluation into VRUs' work are numerous and varied, including:

- **Enhancing accountability.** By providing a mechanism to assess VRUs' performance, evaluation allows stakeholders to hold these units responsible for achieving desired outcomes.
- **Encouraging transparency.** The process of collecting data and reporting findings enables the work of VRUs to be made public, potentially fostering higher levels of trust among stakeholders.
- **Enabling evidence-based decision making.** By helping to generate evidence on the effectiveness of VRUs' work, and the work of those they commission, evaluations can provide solid foundations for informed choices about how to plan and allocate resources in both the short and long term.
- **Sharing best practice.** If made publicly available, evaluations have the potential to ensure efficient and effective practice can be identified and shared across the wider VRU network and beyond.
- **Increasing innovation.** Evaluation can encourage innovative work by highlighting areas where change and improvement are needed.

While these benefits appear to provide a solid rationale for evaluation playing some role in the ongoing development of VRUs, it is worth noting that a number of directors raised concerns about the potential drawbacks associated with evaluation and the reporting it entailed. First, there was a sense that the amount of time and resources being consumed by evaluation and reporting requirements was disproportionate to the potential benefits, and that this burden appeared to be increasing:

> The amount of scrutiny that we've had recently from the Home Office – of various different requests for information, reporting, collation of evidence on top of the usual quarterly reports, the annual report, the strategic needs assessment, the strategy – I think it is becoming a little bit bureaucratic. They want to do a best-practice review at the moment. For me, and I know it's echoed by some of the other directors, if they just pulled the directors together once a quarter, we could share best practice. Instead, we've got to fill out a 40-page document that's extremely repetitive when no one has got the time to do it. (VRU director)

> It's a beast to feed different machines to report back ... I do understand [evaluation] is really important around reassurance to funders, stakeholders, and communities, but I think it is a challenge. It's meeting an expectation that grows and grows and grows. (VRU director)

Related to concerns about the time and resource burdens of collecting, analysing, and compiling data for evaluation reports were anxieties around the possible ethical implications of demanding data on or from young people involved in interventions. Several directors complained about the naivety or indifference of evaluators who seemed to treat data collection as a straightforward technical process, when in reality it concerned sensitive interactions with highly vulnerable children and young people. Some directors were keen to point out that they personally had taken steps to prevent some attempts to gather data on their commissioned interventions, because they thought it was either unnecessary or unethical to collect it:

> I'm the one that stops that piece of paper, that evaluation form, that monitoring form, going out to hardworking grassroots people who are reaching much further than policing can ever do, with a little squeezed-on box that is asking far too much information, certainly that's required by the Home Office, and certainly for us to be able to use it as useful

data. So I am that gatekeeper who's like, 'Why the hell do you want to be asking them that? I'm not sending that out from my unit.' (VRU director)

I've actually got a meeting with the national evaluator next week. But what's happened now twice is that we speak to them, we give them access to our partners, they have conversations, and then last year they said, 'Oh, we'd like to speak to some young people.' I said, 'Whoa, whoa, whoa, I don't want you speaking to any young people because actually we're already running an evaluation speaking to young people, and we're going to have fatigue with all of this going on' ... we're being asked to provide them with young people this year and I just think, no, this started out as programme level, now you're asking about individuals and speaking to young people about their experiences, and actually that's not really what you were set up to do. (VRU director)

Aside from the invasive nature of some data collection being seen as inappropriate, then, some directors were also worried about the potential for evaluations to undermine the potential effectiveness of interventions. This is a commonly reported concern by frontline youth work professionals (see, for example, de St Croix and Doherty, 2022). A further concern was raised in relation to the potential for evaluations to leave intervention participants at an increased risk of harm:

So we had, for example, an issue where it actually created quite a serious safeguarding issue for a young person, because they were found to be consenting to a randomised control trial. They were therefore deemed [by other young people] to be [a police] informant, and so on and so forth. It did create a bit of a safeguarding concern. And it wasn't until we flagged that up to [Organisation A] that there was this acknowledgement eventually that these are real individuals ... also the demands on organisations when

> they receive [Organisation A] funding are huge – the resource that we needed to accommodate it was far more than we ever anticipated. And I certainly know that some VRUs have said they just wouldn't bid in for funding anymore because it's just too much. (VRU director)

As this extract indicates, overly burdensome reporting requirements from evaluators had the potential to prevent VRUs from completing funding applications in the first place. While it may be beneficial from one perspective to increase the amount of data collected in order to better understand the impact of interventions, from another perspective, a disproportionate focus on data collection can pose ethical challenges (for example, in the form of breaching young people's right to privacy and raising potential safeguarding concerns) and undermine the quality and efficacy of interventions (for example, by hindering the smooth functioning of the interventions themselves and reducing the willingness of service providers to apply for funding that comes with burdensome strings attached).

Many directors were sceptical about the ability of evaluations to fully capture the impact associated with an intervention, particularly if it was targeted at primary prevention:

> You'll never know that doing a programme with a pregnant mum, whether that child will go on to live a positive or negative life has been all because of the VRU, or because they happen to have [a] really good friendship group and mum ended up leaving the horrible domestic violence situation she's in, or had a really good role model in dad when he came out of prison and he changed his life – you just can't say. (VRU director)

There was a sense among directors that the evidence for the effectiveness and impact of primary prevention work could never match that associated with interventions operating further downstream, at a tertiary level, where it was possible to identify reductions in violence on a much shorter timeframe. Directors were concerned about the difficulty of running randomised controlled trials to evaluate the impact of primary prevention work, because of the impossibility of building in long enough follow-up periods to capture any potential reductions in serious violence. For example, an intervention that works to support families with very young children and toddlers would not realise any significant reductions in serious violent behaviour until a decade or more into the future. In this context, with organisations such as the YEF (2022) placing a premium on evidence generated by randomised controlled trials, it is clear to see how the toolkit of 'high impact' interventions with a 'high quality' of evidence will be biased towards downstream, tertiary interventions, for which it is more feasible to run randomised controlled trials.

In some sense, this seems to be a case of putting the cart before the horse – instead of VRUs investing in the types of interventions that align well with their local strategic needs assessments, they are pushed towards prioritising interventions that are amenable to the type of evaluation held in highest regard by the 'what works' randomised controlled trial driven paradigm. Seen in this way, the driver of intervention choice becomes the technical feasibility of the preferred evaluation methods, as opposed to the actual potential of the intervention to prevention serious violence (see Stevenson, 2023).

Related to what some directors saw as a disproportionate emphasis on the importance of evidence generated by randomised controlled trials, one interviewee also stressed the importance of factoring in the timeliness of evidence, in addition to the methods by which it was generated:

> If you take a highly evidential approach and how you put that together, first of all, you start going further back into the past … someone's doing a systematic review of systematic reviews and lo and behold, before you've noticed it, you're using papers from 1982, before anyone had a mobile phone, but no one has noticed that. So you've got to have a more relaxed way of looking at it – yes, we need evidence and some things are contemporary and important, but we probably need to relax what we think a little bit more around what strong evidence is. (Professor and NHS consultant)

None of this is to undermine the importance of conducting high-quality evaluations of commissioned interventions. Several directors were keen to highlight the progress made by their VRUs, which were now going beyond simply commissioning violence reduction interventions and 'hoping for the best':

> In 2019, it would be very much getting money out the door and hoping for the best, if we're honest. But as we've grown as a VRU, we've now got a process whereby we take applications, we support grassroots organisations in building theories of change, helping them look at the right data, helping them identify the outcomes that they're looking to impact upon, and then supporting them and partnering them with an evaluator. So, they're not only able to strengthen their own skills and knowledge in terms of evidence-based evaluation, but we're also able to prove impact in terms of what they're delivering, which obviously enables them to leverage funding from other sources. (VRU director)

The VRU mentioned in this extract was seeking to increase the quality of the violence reduction interventions being delivered in its region, as well as increasing their quantity. This is important, because there was a general sense among directors that too many organisations were delivering violence reduction interventions without an adequate understanding of how their work was intended to reduce violence (theories of change), and without the efficacy of these interventions being robustly evaluated.

One common source of frustration among directors concerned the central evaluations of VRUs' own work that were commissioned by the Home Office. Directors reported that these evaluations were taking an unduly long time to publish their findings and recommendations, which sometimes lacked specificity concerning the implications for VRU policy and practice:

> The other thing is that [the Home Office commissioned evaluation team] do their research, then they go away, and we don't hear anything. I mean, I think next week

at the directors' conference we are going to hear about last year's evaluation, but it's just such a long time before we ever hear anything, and then the findings are quite broad and vague, so it's quite difficult to get a sense of any learning from that that we could effectively use. (VRU director)

In summary, then, numerous benefits can flow from high-quality evaluations and reporting. When evaluation is done well, this can support VRUs to invest money in the most impactful and cost-effective violence reduction interventions. Evaluations of VRUs themselves have the potential to generate year-on-year evidence that can help secure continued political support for these units. However, when done badly, evaluations can hinder the work of those delivering interventions and of the VRUs themselves, placing disproportionate time and resource burdens on already stretched organisations. Furthermore, when implemented without sufficient care, evaluations have the potential to raise serious ethical and safeguarding issues, such as in the case of the young person perceived to be a police informant outlined earlier. Instead of supporting and improving protection efforts, poorly designed and badly implemented evaluations have the potential to undermine engagement, and place children and young people at an increased risk of harm.

Influencing government and institutional policies

VRUs' role in enhancing multi-agency collaboration, engaging with young people and communities, and commissioning timely and effective programmatic interventions, are three important strands of current violence prevention efforts in England and Wales. What remains, however, is a vast range of governmental and institutional policies that influence, transform, and, in certain cases, constrain the lives of children and young people. Although they are rarely perceived in terms of violence prevention, it is clear that these policies – for example, housing policy, welfare policy, educational policy, and economic policy – play a pivotal role in shaping young people's mental and physical health, the relationships they experience, and the opportunities open to them to pursue fulfilling and meaningful lives. Effective violence prevention strategies, therefore, must be expansive and take into account the extent to which such policies are likely to reduce or exacerbate rates of violence.

Before turning to the work of VRUs in England and Wales, it is worth briefly reflecting on the role of the Scottish VRU in this area. The Scottish VRU was, initially, a small team of police officers and analysts with significant freedom to experiment and innovate. During our interviews, members of the Scottish VRU recalled the early years as 'a bit of the Wild West', 'very organic' and 'quite instantaneous'. New ideas were developed and tested at pace, and discarded or altered accordingly. Arguably, one of the most successful contributions of the Scottish VRU was its role as an influencer across multiple areas of national and institutional policy. The Scottish VRU worked both horizontally – seeking to enhance work between agencies, gather a 'coalition of the willing', and build a cross-sector movement for change – and vertically, investing time and energy in reshaping national policy. This is because it recognised that the root causes of violence lay not with individuals, but in the wider systems and structures that shaped their lives.

When talking about the perceived success of the Scottish VRU, many VRU directors in England and Wales spoke about the importance of change at a national policy level:

> For me, I think it was the wider changes in policy, so around alcohol policy, social housing policy, so it was a truly system-wide approach, rather than just tinkering around the edges. (VRU director)

> I think we have to get a stronger voice around inequality and I think, to some extent, the Scottish VRU does this quite well and it has really highlighted the link between poverty and inequality and violence, but I think we need to get much better at that and shouting about it from the rooftops and really understanding how to, kind of, utilise public health approaches in the violence prevention space to properly address inequality ... not just socioeconomic inequality, but racial inequality and gender inequality. (VRU director)

The-then United Kingdom (UK) Home Secretary, Sajid Javid, and regional mayors such as Sadiq Khan and Andy Burnham, have all expressed their desire for the public health approach to violence prevention in England and Wales to be inspired and informed by lessons from north of the border (see Mayor of London, 2018; Wright and Hughes, 2018; Mayor of Greater Manchester, 2023). During our interviews, VRU directors themselves often framed the Scottish VRU as a model to learn from. Work to influence national-level policy, however, was generally regarded as a key shortcoming of the VRUs in England and Wales during their early years of operation, despite it being something that directors generally aspired to do. Among the reasons for this shortcoming was the perceived trap of overspending and overfocusing on commissioned interventions, at the expense of VRU staff time and resources being directed towards national and institutional policy change:

> I think because of the nature of commissioning, it can keep you there as well, quite quickly, because it's such an industry, isn't it? I know across the VRU network nationally there are some areas that spent like 80–90 per cent of their budget on commissioning services ... when grant money comes in, it's quite unusual to spend it on anything other than commissioning services ... I do want a chunk, it was about 50 per cent of our budget, I do want it spent on staff, on doers, people to actually do things. I know other areas didn't make that decision, and as a result, they really struggled to keep that balance between the different principles of a public health approach. (VRU director)

For many directors, although there was a desire to replicate the successful policy engagement work of the Scottish VRU, they perceived themselves to be hampered by the fact that this activity was less capable of generating quick political capital relative to the 'sparkle' and 'glitz' of newly commissioned interventions:

> I know that other directors felt the pressure a lot more than we did to spend money on new things

like new interventions. I mean, just to give you an example, after about four weeks of existence, a senior stakeholder saw me in a corridor somewhere and said, 'We need more sparkle, we need more glitz, we need something that's going to, you know?' And it's trying to kind of resist that, let's just spend money on a sparkly project that's going to look good in a newsletter, or on Twitter, or whatever. (VRU director)

In addition to the pull of 'sparkly projects', there were certain pushes that steered senior managers away from substantive engagement with national and institutional policy change:

There is something around needing to see a result and needing to see a result quickly ... there's something around, you get five years maximum of government, before you change, so, therefore, you know, what can we do within a term of parliament? What can be delivered? ... it's a lot easier, therefore, within those time constraints, and those funding constraints, to do something that's a short-term programme ... rather than going right back to the institutions and then I think it comes back to that point around, actually, people think it's too big. And my argument, again, is, actually, it's not too big if you break it down and cut through it, and look at what is actually needed, and then you can see that there are pathways and ways forward. (Senior staff member, Youth Justice Board)

Finally, and to return to the point about the importance of evaluations in shaping the work of VRUs made earlier in this chapter, there was a perception that VRU time and resources directed at the level of policy change would likely not be recognised adequately in evaluations:

The Home Office are now far more interested in numbers of young people engaged, and that really started to ramp up last year. And that leads you to commissioning services that are simply engaging with individual young people. Whereas some of the approaches we've taken, if I pick schools, for example, we've had two projects running, one with some mainstream secondary schools about changing the approach to inclusion, and that's working with the school professionals, it's about their policy and practice ... we can't report on that to the Home Office because they've really been focused on counting bums on seats. But I think I would argue that actually, in terms of things like education, if you change the culture of the educational establishment, if you upskill the staff, you are going to have that much longer-term impact. (VRU director)

Despite these challenges, many directors clearly had an appetite to pursue government- and institutional-level policy change, with one director suggesting that the Serious Violence Duty provided a 'good gateway' into this type of work:

[Through the Duty] we've been able to further build our understanding of the scale of youth violence and the root causes, which is great, but the more datasets you have, it tells the same story: that you need to stop harming young people, and they'll be less harmful when they grow up ... the Serious Violence Duty then gives us that opportunity to influence policy, because we know the policies that we've got in place locally and nationally, they don't stop harming children, so it's a good gateway into that. (VRU director)

The argument being made here is that the more data that is shared and analysed, the clearer it becomes that certain government and institutional policies are likely to be exacerbating rates of serious violence. These include, for example, successive government housing policies that have resulted in tens of thousands of young people living in inadequate and insecure accommodation (Ministry of Housing, Communities and Local Government, 2024), or educational policies that result in tens of thousands of young people being subject to extended periods of isolation in schools, or suspensions and exclusions (Children's Commissioner, 2019).

Despite the challenges outlined here, a number of directors spoke about their progress in influencing government and institutional policies:

> In terms of influencing government policy, this probably isn't reflected as strongly in our priorities. But certainly, I see that as a key responsibility for us. So, one of the things that we've done in [Area A] was to [support Person B] in the change to the Serious Violence Duty scope. So there was an event at the House of Lords in September 2021 I think that was to ensure that sexual violence and domestic violence was included in the scope of serious violence. And so certainly, there's things we've done. And we're also part of the Hope Collective, as a lot of VRUs are. (VRU director)

The Hope Collective referred to in this extract describes itself as a movement to bring together groups and individuals who wish to work together to 'influence policy making' and 'establish real change', aimed primarily at reducing poverty, violence, and discrimination in UK communities (Hope Collective, 2022b). It is telling that the vast majority of VRUs in England and Wales had committed their support and engagement to the Hope Collective, with many co-organising and hosting events described as 'Hope Hacks', designed to bring young people together to discuss the sort of society they would like to grow up in, and the types of policy change that might be needed to bring those visions about. At the time of writing, the Hope Collective had run over 30 Hope Hacks across the UK, attended by more than 3,000 young people (Rennie, 2024).

The London VRU in particular has had some success in influencing institutional policies. In part, this is due to the fact that its funding far exceeds that of the other regional VRUs. While the London VRU receives more money from the Home Office than any other VRU, it also receives an even greater sum from the Mayor of London (Mayor of London, 2022). The political backing the unit receives from the Mayor also enhances its potential clout at the level of national and institutional policy making. Moving beyond their commissioning and multi-agency working functions, the London VRU has made notable strides in influencing school policy in the region. In what has come to be known as 'London's Inclusion Charter', the VRU led a partnership approach that combined the voices of young people, teachers, parents and carers, local authorities, and education specialists. The purpose of the charter is to promote inclusive practices in London's schools, intended to reduce absenteeism and the suspension and exclusion of pupils (London Violence Reduction Unit, 2024).

In this case, the London VRU acted on its strategic needs assessment and evidence that suggested a close link between school exclusions and increased rates of violence between young people (see, for example, APPG Knife Crime, 2019; Irwin-Rogers et al, 2020; Cathro et al, 2023). The unit worked with an important institution in young people's lives (in this case, schools) to enhance the safety and wellbeing of pupils. It is vital to note, however, that the success of this initiative is to some extent contingent on national policies and agencies – were the Department for Education and Ofsted to advance complementary guidance, for instance, this would substantially increase the likelihood of reducing levels of school exclusion (Billingham and Gillon, 2024). This is another example, then, of the urgent need for national-level change to complement the work of regional VRUs. Particularly given VRUs' limited powers over crucial sectors such as education, the regional efforts of VRUs should be better supported by government action at a national level, undertaken in dialogue with VRUs.

Conclusion

This chapter has completed our exploration of the work of regional VRUs in England and Wales. It focused first on VRUs' role as commissioners of violence reduction interventions. All VRUs were spending a sizeable proportion of their budget on interventions, with directors viewing this strand of their work as vital to the overall success of their violence prevention efforts. Challenges arose, however, over the extent to which directors felt able to invest in interventions at the level of primary prevention – that is, upstream work that aims to prevent violence over the long term. Barriers to primary prevention included narrow performance metrics and pressure from key stakeholders, both of which demanded short-term impact. Moreover, although there was an abundance of delivery organisations offering interventions at the secondary and tertiary levels, some directors reported that high-quality primary-level interventions were relatively scarce, making it difficult to scale up this type of work. In addition, while directors were keen to scale up effective interventions, they pointed to declining year-on-year budgets that made this process difficult.

A major theme that directors were keen to discuss at length was the role and significance of evaluations and reporting. When evaluations were done well, they provided an important source of guidance that helped directors to decide where to focus their resources. However, too often evaluations imposed what were perceived to be disproportionate reporting requirements on delivery organisations, and generated reports that were ambiguous in their implications.

The chapter then considered the extent to which VRUs had been successful in influencing national and institutional policies that shape children and young people's lives and make up the broader landscape of violence prevention. Most directors were keen for their VRUs to play an important role here, but at the same time they acknowledged this was an area where their units were currently falling short. Reasons for this included the fact that VRU resources were limited, particularly in relation to the size of the task – there are many competing and powerful forces that drag national and institutional policies in different directions, making them difficult to influence. Nevertheless, the largest and most well funded of the VRU network, the London VRU, had made some progress, most notably in the area of education. This indicates the importance not only of adequate levels of funding, but also of high-level political backing for VRUs (which the London VRU received from the Mayor of London), if regional VRUs are to fulfil their potential in advancing a truly holistic public health approach to violence prevention.

In the final chapter, we expand our scope to consider the public health approach to violence prevention more broadly, addressing the critical question: Where should we go from here?

PART III
Looking ahead

5

Where should we go from here?

So far, this book has provided a history of the public health approach to violence prevention (Part I), and considered in particular the work of regional Violence Reduction Units (VRUs) in England and Wales (Part II). In this final chapter, we switch to a forward-looking lens and focus on the question: 'Where should we go from here?' We consider this specifically in relation to the work of VRUs, but also in relation to the public health approach to violence prevention more broadly. While we contend that VRUs can play an important role in advancing public health approaches in the years ahead, there are things that need to be done above and beyond the work of VRUs if we are to secure a safer society for children and young people in the long term.

The chapter consists of six sections. In the first section, we revisit and expand on the 'Four Is' framework that featured briefly in the Introduction to this book. In the second section, we apply the Four Is framework to recent violence prevention initiatives, to explore the ways in which these initiatives have sought to achieve change at the levels of inequalities, institutions, interventions, and interactions.

In the third section, we return to our conceptualisation of a holistic public health approach to violence prevention, explaining how it relates to and is enriched by the Four Is framework. We also briefly discuss international comparative research on the societal determinants of violence, in order to further substantiate our belief in the need for a public health approach that operates at all four levels of the Four Is framework.

In the fourth section, we discuss the future of VRUs, in light of the findings and arguments we presented in previous chapters, as well as in the context of the Four Is framework. In the fifth section, we outline some of the potential limitations and pitfalls associated with the arguments made in this book. Finally, in the sixth section, we conclude the chapter.

Our central argument in this concluding chapter is that a truly holistic public health approach to violence prevention should entail coordinated and complementary work at four interconnected levels: the levels of inequalities, institutions, interventions, and interactions.

Preventing violence through coordinated action across the Four Is

Based on the findings of the 'Public Health, Youth and Violence Reduction' (PHYVR) project as whole, we believe a Four Is framework is useful for advancing a more effective public health approach to violence prevention in England and Wales (see Figure 6 in the Introduction).

Before we look more specifically at the effects of recent violence prevention initiatives on these Four Is, we first provide some context by briefly presenting a sketched 'state of the nation' report in relation to each 'I'.

Inequalities in society

At the macro level of inequalities, it is impossible to overlook the United Kingdom's (UK's) highly unequal distribution of wealth and income. The UK ranks as the eighth most unequal of the 37 countries of the Organisation for Economic Co-operation and Development (OECD), as measured by the Gini coefficient (OECD, 2023). The number of children living in relative poverty in the UK (after housing costs) was 4.3 million in 2022/23 (Child Poverty Action Group, 2024a). Brewer et al (2023) forecast that relative child poverty will continue to increase and reach its highest levels on record in 2027–28. In practical terms, millions of children in the UK find themselves living in insecure and inadequate accommodation, with their families unable to afford bills, food, and other basic household items.

Inequalities in income and wealth are accompanied by other forms of inequality and social injustice, including class and racial prejudice. In relation to the former, there is no shortage of examples of people with the least wealth and income being stigmatised and discriminated against (see, for example, Tyler, 2020). In relation to the latter, a range of social statistics, as well as first-hand accounts, demonstrate the persistence of abuse and discrimination that many UK citizens face on the basis of their perceived 'race' (Byrne et al, 2020). From police stop and search, to sentencing, to youth custody, to the adult prison estate, the criminal justice system has a disproportionate impact on low-income and racialised populations (see, for example, Williams and Clarke, 2018; Prison Reform Trust, 2021).

All of these inequalities increase the likelihood of young people committing acts of serious violence by engendering structural humiliation among those who are worst affected, amplifying the levels of shame and stigma they experience and undermining their sense of mattering. In this regard, it is important to stress that explanation is not exoneration. Recognising that different ways of organising and structuring societies will generate more or less violence does not mean that individuals can or should be absolved of blame and responsibility for their actions. If a young person commits an act of violence, they can and should be held appropriately accountable.[1] However, this does not change the fact that if we wish to bring about safer societies, we cannot neglect to address significant inequalities that currently exist in the UK, and in many other countries around the world.

Institutions, services, and social infrastructure

There are many glaring problems affecting the institutions, services, and social infrastructure in the UK that should help to keep children safe. This can be exemplified by a handful of cases. Youth services, for instance, have been decimated since 2010, including through the closure of many long-running youth centres, which were embedded in communities and provided support to young people through multiple generations (Weale, 2020). The rates and consequences of school exclusions and suspensions are also a cause for deep concern, particularly in England, with permanent exclusions rising towards pre-pandemic levels, and suspensions at their highest levels since 2006 (Department for Education, 2024). The Children's Commissioner (2019), among others, has highlighted the connections between school exclusions and risk of violence.

Flaws and failures in children's custodial settings are entrenched and chronic – in light of the 2022/23 *Children in Custody* annual report (HMIP, 2023, p 3), the Chief Inspector of Prisons said that 'the Youth Custody Service are unable to guarantee basic services for children'. The number of children in temporary accommodation doubled between 2011 and 2023 (Ministry of Housing, Communities and Local Government, 2023), and the rate of young men aged 16–24 not in education, employment or training in England and Wales rose from 9 per cent in 2000 to 13 per cent in 2024 (Office for National Statistics, 2024c). Our children's social care system has experienced heightened need and reduced resources over the past decade (Hood et al, 2020). Thus, for many of our children and young people, and particularly the most vulnerable, our institutions and services are failing to provide the most basic building blocks for safety and wellbeing.

Interventions and programmes

We use the terms 'interventions' and 'programmes' to refer broadly to more-or-less well-defined and delineated sets of bounded activity, which are designed to achieve certain outcomes with a particular target individual or group, often over a set time period. This can include mentoring projects designed to boost young people's aspirations, for instance, or parenting classes intended to enhance parental capacities. There is a wide array of interventions and programmes being delivered across England and Wales to support children and young people, parents, and families, to address a range of different needs and capacities. These interventions take place in a number of settings, including community centres, schools, healthcare settings, children's centres, and through home visits. They are funded through a variety of sources, including central and local government, and philanthropic trusts and foundations. There is a burgeoning 'what works' movement compiling evaluations that evidence the (in)effectiveness of programmatic interventions, including the Early Intervention Foundation, the Educational Endowment Fund, the Youth Futures Foundation, and – as discussed throughout this book, and further later in this chapter, the Youth Endowment Fund (YEF).

The benefits of high-quality interventions can be substantial (as highlighted by the 'what works' centres mentioned earlier), and the demand for such interventions can be significant, among central and local governments, particular institutions such as schools, and among children, young people, and families themselves. Interventions can be a highly effective and efficient means to address well-identified needs and issues. There is a debate, however, about the overall societal effect of interventions: while some researchers suggest that an accumulation of efficacious interventions can deliver significant beneficial social change (Wilson et al, 2024), others argue that interventions more often achieve patchy and short-lived societal improvements, particularly relative to more systematic or structural changes (Stevenson, 2023). Relatedly, it has been argued that an overreliance on high-profile, well-promoted interventions can distract and detract from the urgent need for change at the levels of our two preceding 'Is': inequalities and institutions. Indeed, two of the authors of this book have contributed to a paper that makes this argument in relation to the 'state of play' in the criminal justice system in England and Wales, highlighting the dangers of the propensity among policy makers to favour (sometimes flawed and harmful) interventions over more fundamental changes to institutions, services, systems, and policies – a propensity that we label 'interventionitis' (Stevens et al, 2025).

Interactions and relationships

The inequalities and institutional inadequacies that we have discussed have direct consequences for the quality of relationships in children and young people's lives, whether with family, friends, or adult professionals. Inequalities and discrimination affect personal and professional relationships of all kinds. Some of the institutional issues outlined earlier shape relationships in a variety of ways:

- many young people have lost access to supportive youth work relationships, or are only able to have very superficial relationships with helping professionals, including social workers, due to their excessive caseloads (Ravalier et al, 2021; National Youth Agency, 2024);
- housing issues exacerbate family tensions and can result in relocation away from community networks (Hock et al, 2024);
- school exclusions often abruptly separate young people from their friendship groups (Arnez and Condry, 2021).

Heightened demand for children's social care services in England and Wales over the past decade is, in part, a reflection of these relational deficits.

High-quality interventions and programmes are often intended to provide or enhance supportive relationships in children and young people's lives, but in worst cases, if designed or implemented badly, they can result in tarnished relationships. Brierley (2021) has coined the term 'relational poverty' to describe the acute scarcity of supportive relationships in many young people's lives, suggesting that there is a close connection between this experience and the perpetration of violent behaviour.

Recent violence prevention initiatives: applying a Four Is lens

In this section, we consider the successes and shortcomings, strengths and weaknesses of recent violence prevention policy initiatives in England and Wales by discussing their (potential) effects on the Four Is. In so doing, we summarise many of the key arguments that we have advanced throughout this book. We focus on the three key initiatives that have been most prominently associated with the public health approach by the UK government (see Chapter 2): VRUs, the YEF, and the Serious Violence Duty.

Violence Reduction Units

Part II of this book looked squarely and in-depth at the work of VRUs, so we will provide only a brief recap here. Based on our interviews with all of the regional VRUs in England and Wales, it is clear that they have been taking a multi-pronged approach to preventing violence, which includes:

- enhancing multi-agency working and data sharing;
- commissioning and evaluating interventions to prevent and reduce violence;
- listening to and amplifying the voices of communities and young people to better inform responses to violence.

Annual evaluations of the work of VRUs have already generated some evidence of success in reducing violence in their respective regions (Home Office, 2023). The same evaluations have highlighted the effective work of VRUs in pushing the issue of violence up the list of priorities of various agencies with a stake in safeguarding young people. During our interviews, VRU directors were keen to talk about the progress their units have made in bringing organisations together to collaborate on the issue of violence prevention and the positive impact of many of the programmatic interventions their units had commissioned. Despite this progress, challenges remain. VRUs have struggled to develop long-term violence prevention strategies that tackle the root causes of violence, or that attempt to address some of the major societal inequalities that adversely impact the lives of so many children and young people. Narrow performance metrics, pressure from various stakeholders with vested interests in securing immediate results, and short-term funding arrangements, have all undermined the ability of VRUs to pursue long-term, primary prevention.

The Youth Endowment Fund

As touched upon throughout this book, the YEF exists to fund and evaluate violence reduction interventions, and was established in 2019 with £200 million of Home Office funding. The YEF has invested considerable resources in the production of a 'toolkit' that summarises evidence on a wide range of violence reduction interventions, based on findings from over 2,000 studies. Each of the 20 regional VRUs in England and Wales is mandated to spend at least 20 per cent of its budget on the commissioning of interventions that are identified by the YEF toolkit as 'high impact'. The latest evaluation of VRUs showed that a total of 327 violence reduction interventions were commissioned by these units during 2022/23, supporting an estimated 271,783 young people (Home Office, 2023). These are significant numbers, and it is clear from the evaluation that many children and young people are likely to have benefited in various ways from this work – particularly where these interventions have provided them with new or enhanced supportive relationships.

More recently, the YEF has begun to produce 'systems guidance', outlining potential changes to protocols and approaches that could make a positive difference at specific points of certain institutions, systems, and services (our second 'I') such as point of arrest (YEF, 2023). And in April 2024, the YEF released an application for the post of 'research lead: underlying causes of violence' – a clear declaration of intent that their work is set to expand beyond its earlier relatively narrow focus on programmatic interventions, to include an exploration of the effects of societal inequalities (YEF, 2024b).

YEF can thus be seen to have developed work across all four 'Is'. Returning to the point about 'inteventionitis' outlined earlier, however, YEF's principal focus on promoting interventions arguably constrains its ability to encourage more fundamental institutional, systemic, and societal changes, nudging the attention of policy makers and commissioners instead towards short-term interventions and programmes.

The Serious Violence Duty

The Serious Violence Duty (the Duty), which came into force in 2023, has prompted existing services to work more closely together to support and safeguard children and young people. This is important, because organisations working in silos are liable to reduce the efficiency and effectiveness of all services (Public Health

England, 2019). Many VRU directors were keen to highlight the value of the Duty in bringing relevant stakeholders onto the same page. Our interviewees raised concerns about increasingly stretched agencies, however. The services subject to the Duty – the police, youth offending teams, local authorities, local health boards, integrated care boards, fire and rescue authorities, and probation – currently find themselves struggling under the weight of increasing demand and depleted resources, after a long period of austerity in public services. There is a limit as to what can be achieved by enhancing collaboration between agencies experiencing acute resource scarcity.

In summary, then, while recent policy initiatives go some way towards advancing efforts at violence prevention, they constitute piecemeal steps that neglect important drivers of violence at the macro level of societal inequalities and institutions. Without further action being taken at a national policy level across various areas of social policy, these recent initiatives are unlikely to shift the dial on many of the entrenched root causes of violence. To bring about a safer society, a wider-ranging and more ambitious vision is needed along the lines of that originally envisaged by those attending the United States (US) Surgeon General workshop on violence and public health almost four decades ago (US Department of Health and Human Services, 1986, discussed in Chapter 1).

Advancing a truly holistic public health approach to violence prevention

To go beyond these existing policy measures, then, and for England and Wales to become and remain a permanently low-violence society, we should make a strong and enduring commitment to a truly holistic public health approach to violence prevention, which would consist of wide-ranging activities addressing each level of the 'Four I's. Expanding on the three-principle conceptualisation outlined in the Introduction to this book, we consider there to be four key principles of a holistic public health approach:

- **levels of activity – 'the what':** recognising that violence is best understood as the product of particular factors operating at the societal, community, familial, and individual levels, which

can only be addressed through coordinated activity across the levels of all Four Is;
- **stages of prevention – 'the when':** ensuring that efforts to prevent violence involve an appropriate balance of work at the primary, secondary, and tertiary levels, through both universal and targeted provision;
- **model of implementation – 'the how':** following the World Health Organization's (WHO's) four-step model: (i) defining and mapping the problem of violence; (ii) identifying the causes of violence; (iii) designing, implementing, and evaluating policies and interventions to find out what works to prevent violence; and (iv) embedding and expanding policies and scaling up interventions that work;
- **central, regional, and local government action – 'the where':** ensuring that complementary violence prevention activity takes place at the central, regional, and local levels.[2]

In theory, these four principles are coherent and complementary. In practice, however, an inappropriately narrow interpretation of the model of implementation ('the how') has the potential to undermine the other three. The problem here, as we see it, is that the term 'interventions' has often been interpreted narrowly to mean 'programmatic interventions operating at a local or community level'. A narrow interpretation thereby excludes other preventative efforts such as national-level policy change that could equally be (but is typically not) regarded as an 'intervention'. Specifically, then, we would refine the aims of the WHO's model of implementation as follows:

- to define the problem through the systematic collection of information about the magnitude, scope, characteristics, and consequences of violence;
- to establish why violence occurs using research to determine the causes and correlates of violence, the factors that increase or decrease the risk of violence, and the factors that could be modified through interventions;
- to find out what works to prevent violence by designing, implementing, and evaluating *national and regional policies and programmatic* interventions;

- to implement effective and promising *policies and programmatic* interventions in a wide range of settings – the effects of these *policies and programmatic* interventions on risk factors and the target outcomes should be monitored, and their impact and cost-effectiveness should be evaluated.

Our proposed revision would encourage a vision of the public health approach to violence prevention that involves all three types of prevention (where currently in practice it focuses predominantly on secondary and tertiary prevention), and that operates at all four levels of the ecological framework (where currently in practice it operates predominantly at the levels of community, family, and the individual).

In short, a commitment to the four core principles of a truly holistic public health approach to violence prevention would mean:

- addressing the causes of violence that operate at different levels;
- providing effective universal prevention, targeted interventions for those at-risk, and support and rehabilitation for those already involved in serious violence;
- systematically developing and implementing effective programmatic interventions and policies;
- ensuring that central, regional, and local governments embrace their share of responsibility for bringing about safer societies.

In relation to the last of these, without action at a central government level – something that we argue is sorely lacking in present-day England and Wales – VRUs and other regional and local agencies risk becoming overly responsibilised for the task of preventing violence, and perpetually grappling with the local manifestations of problems that need to be addressed by central government at a national level.

One of the major limitations associated with the current approach to violence prevention in England and Wales is that its gaze is directed disproportionately at the level of programmatic interventions, which locate the problem of violence in the attitudes and behaviour of 'at-risk' individuals. To be clear, VRU and YEF attempts to fund and scale up programmatic interventions are one important strand in any violence prevention strategy, particularly at regional and local levels. However, this has the potential to distract from important work that must take place at the macro level of societal inequalities and institutions – work that is needed to provide the basic building blocks of safety and wellbeing for all our children and young people. One of our interviewees captured this point well:

> Earlier this week I was in a meeting … about addressing social determinants *or* individual family and community-level interventions. And the answer is you clearly need both – please stop arguing about whether you need one or the other. I could go on and fill the whole hour with why you need both. But you not only need both, you also need people who represent both to work together. (Professor and NHS consultant)

Addressing societal inequalities and improving the quality of key institutions is a complex challenge and various perspectives exist on how this can be achieved in modern societies. Some, including Winlow and Hall (2022), argue for extensive transformation of capitalist political economies. Others, such as Reich (2016) and Piketty (2020), advocate for significant yet less radical reforms. Still others, including Ridley (2011) and Norberg (2016), broadly defend the status quo, emphasising the merits of existing forms of political economy.

Regardless of one's position in these debates, we contend that to understand and effectively address violence, we cannot neglect the fundamental role of societal inequalities and institutions, both of which play crucial roles in shaping children and young people's lives. Yet, policy makers too often remain silent on these issues, focusing instead on the potential of programmatic interventions to solve the problem of violence. This must change moving forwards if we are to secure a society with permanently low levels of violence.

The type of policy implications that flow from these conclusions include, among other things:

- ensuring our schools are well resourced and staffed by teachers who are valued, adequately trained, paid fairly, and have decent working conditions;
- enhancing youth work provision, recognising it as a vital source of support, and reversing a decade of deep cuts and neglect;
- rapidly expanding the provision of decent and affordable homes to tackle rising rates of homelessness and housing insecurity;
- establishing robust and high-quality systems of child and family support;
- developing a youth justice system that genuinely serves the interests of children, young people, and society as a whole.[3]

Securing a safer society will require a bold and ambitious programme of change across a range of social policy areas.

Learning lessons from a global perspective

Zooming out to a global perspective can also help to strengthen the case for a holistic public health approach to violence prevention, which delivers changes across the Four Is. Taking a global perspective and drawing on an extensive body of international evidence, Currie (2016) substantiated the WHO model, concluding that societies with low rates of violence tend to:

- adopt social policies that produce low levels of socioeconomic inequality;
- avoid harsh and ineffective criminal justice systems that serve to exacerbate root causes and perpetuate cycles of violence;
- provide strong social supports, including family support programmes, high-quality and accessible mental health services, and family-friendly economic policies;
- make it difficult for people to access firearms;
- minimise levels of marginal work (jobs that are demeaning and very low paid) and maximise the availability of inclusive forms of work (jobs that allow people to make a decent living and foster a sense of purpose and self-worth).

Importantly, there are few (if any) examples of countries that have undergone significant and sustained reductions in violence through the implementation of programmatic interventions (see further Stevenson, 2023). To reiterate, this does not mean that interventions cannot form part of an effective violence prevention strategy. However, it is important to ensure that a focus on localised interventions does not crowd out efforts to address the deep-rooted societal and community drivers of violence. In other words, effective violence prevention requires mutually supportive and coordinated work across all four levels of the Four Is framework.

Before we conclude, given the focus on VRUs in Part II of this book, it is worth focusing squarely on the potential direction of travel for these units in the years ahead.

The future of Violence Reduction Units

At the time of writing, many VRU directors reported feeling uncertain about the long-term future of their units. Given the early progress and success of VRUs – as discussed at length in Part II of this book and evidenced in formal yearly evaluations (see Home Office, 2022c, 2023c, 2023d) – we hope to see the Home Office continuing to support and invest in these units in the coming years. As part of a face-to-face workshop the PHYVR team hosted with VRU directors in September 2023, we discussed, among other things, the possible future of VRUs in England and Wales. For VRUs to best contribute to the advancement of a holistic public health approach to violence prevention, we share here some key recommendations based on the findings from our interviews and workshops.

Local coordination of, and encouragement for, joined-up working

VRUs play a valuable role in galvanising and coordinating regional and local agencies to collaborate closely in their efforts to prevent violence. They work in tandem with local authorities and with high-level multi-agency bodies such as community safety partnerships, local safeguarding boards, and integrated commissioning boards to ensure that high-quality violence prevention activities are occurring in their areas, in line with each of the 'what', 'when' and 'how' principles outlined in our conceptualisation of the public health approach. VRUs often play a key role in the multi-agency arrangements for violence reduction mandated by the Serious Violence Duty, for instance. In London, the VRU works with all of the city's local authorities on tailored 'violence and vulnerability plans' for each borough. These plans provide a means through which the VRU can provide dedicated support (and challenge) to enhance violence reduction efforts across the capital.

Improving evaluation criteria

It is clearly proving difficult for VRUs to get upstream of the problem of violence and focus their resources and attention on early intervention. This undermines their ability to adhere to the second core principle of the public health approach outlined earlier – that it should involve a well-balanced mix of activities at each stage of prevention (primary, secondary, and tertiary). To some extent, as discussed in Chapter 4, this is because directors perceive themselves to be under significant pressure to achieve quick wins in terms of reductions in violence. One source of pressure stems from the annual VRU evaluations, which use the following two 'primary outcome' metrics to draw conclusions about the success or failure of VRUs: homicides and hospital admissions for injury by a sharp object. While there is an obvious rationale for using these metrics as part of VRU evaluations, there are two important objections worth raising.

First, there are many other metrics and criteria by which VRUs might be evaluated – and many which VRU directors themselves thought would constitute more appropriate 'primary outcomes'. The final session of our VRU director workshop addressed the question: 'What does a good VRU look like?' The room was split into six tables, with each being asked to identify the most and least appropriate metrics for evaluating the quality and success of VRUs' work. By far the most popular proposed criterion for evaluating VRU success was 'feelings of safety among children and young people' (see the Appendix for full results of the activity). For various reasons, including the objection discussed earlier, the current primary outcome measures failed to make the top ten list of any of the six groups completing the activity.

Second, as acknowledged in the annual evaluations themselves, the two primary outcomes (homicides and hospital admissions for injury by a sharp object) are 'low count' outcomes (that is, there are relatively few incidents per year, compared with other forms of violence with less severe injury). This makes it exceptionally difficult for VRUs to generate reductions in these outcomes that will reach the required level of statistical significance. As such (and in every annual evaluation to date), the conclusion drawn is that VRUs have had 'no statistically significant impact on the primary serious violence outcomes' (Home Office, 2023c). Unfortunately, there is clear potential for this result to be misinterpreted by readers (including policy makers) who may take it to mean that VRUs have had no impact on homicides or sharp-object hospital admissions. What the result actually means, however, is that there is too much natural variance/noise in the data to be confident that the change in the (low-count) primary outcome variables can be attributed to the impact of VRUs. Indeed, it seems likely that, given the level of nature variance/noise in the data, annual evaluations could run for the next one hundred years, and none would ever find results on these primary outcome measures that would reach the level of statistical significance.

This is a relic of rules associated with current forms of statistical analysis, rather than representing anything meaningful about the work of VRUs. Simply put, the complexity of the social world is such that we cannot with sufficient confidence say whether or not VRU activity is impacting on these primary outcomes – a reflection of our limited ability to make sense of the social world, rather than of an absence of VRU impact per se.

To help ensure that VRUs provide sufficient resources and attention to upstream violence prevention efforts, it would be helpful for VRU evaluations to give greater emphasis to other outcomes, including, but not limited to, children and young people's feelings of safety. And, in accordance with the analysis in Part II of this book, it would be useful if government ministers, police and crime commissioners and other key stakeholders struck an appropriate balance between the imperatives of long-term primary prevention and short-term secondary and tertiary violence reduction.

Foregrounding the social and economic drivers of violence

One of the main successes of VRUs to date has been in pushing the issue of violence prevention up the agendas of various partner agencies. As discussed earlier, VRUs now play a pivotal role in the implementation of the Serious Violence Duty. However, too often, multi-agency partnerships pursue an approach to safeguarding that focuses predominantly on changing individual behaviour, as opposed to improving environments and social conditions. A recent study by Owens and Lloyd (2023), for example, found an absence of ecological approaches in multi-agency partnerships – that is, approaches that essentially adhere to the philosophy of contextual safeguarding in addressing the social environments that foster harm, rather than just individual harmful behaviours (see Firmin, 2020). Moving forwards – and particularly given that their local strategic needs assessments serve to identify the social and economic drivers of violence in their respective regions – VRUs could play an important role in redressing this state of affairs by ensuring multi-agency partnerships move beyond narrow approaches to safeguarding that target only individual behaviour, to also address structural problems, such as housing issues, poverty, and access to education and employment.

Moving beyond interventions and multi-agency working

As evidenced in our interviews and discussed at length in Chapters 3 and 4, VRUs in England and Wales have made considerable progress in the commissioning of high-quality violence reduction interventions and in bringing about improved multi-agency working. However, it is important to recognise that the potential value of VRUs extends beyond these two activities. In the case of the Scottish VRU, this unit had considerable success in changing public discourse around violence, as well as the way institutions framed and responded to the problem of violence (Fraser and Gillon, 2023). It is clear that VRUs in England and Wales are currently adopting a somewhat different approach to the task of violence prevention. One interviewee put it as follows:

> I would refrain from saying that England and Wales followed the Scottish example – I don't think they did. I think [VRUs in England and Wales] have similar, strangely, objectives [to the Scottish VRU], but they are based in philosophically different approaches. So what's come out in England has been very, I'd say, too heavily evidenced based – percentages of what each VRU has to do stipulated according to particular evidence ... whereas the Scottish example was much more about advocacy, a call to action, and stuff like that. (Professor and NHS consultant)

The reasons for the divergence between the approach taken by the Scottish VRU compared with VRUs in England and Wales include:

- the regional scope of the units in England and Wales, which contrasts to the national scope of the Scottish VRU;
- the size of the governments operating out of Westminster and Holyrood (the former being much larger than the latter);
- the differing modes of public governance and Westminster's relative embrace of New Public Management principles (see Chapter 4; Fraser et al, forthcoming);
- the remit and evaluation criteria laid out by the Home Office that guide the approach taken by the VRUs in England and Wales.

The London VRU stands out somewhat from the rest of the network on this issue, with this unit enjoying some success in influencing the policies of some key institutions (see Chapter 4). On the whole, however, the regional structure of VRUs in England and Wales and the political context in within which they operate make it relatively challenging for these units to influence national and institutional policies that shape the lives of children and young people.

Long-term funding and support

For VRUs to fulfil their potential, they require long-term funding and support from central and (where feasible) regional governments. The shift from year-on-year funding settlements to a three-year funding settlement was a positive step, but it still leaves VRUs without long-term security and makes it difficult for these units to create long-term (for example, ten-year) plans that their own staff and external partner agencies can feel inspired and confident about. Were VRUs to secure long-term commitments concerning funding and support, it would provide a degree of confidence within the network that has been lacking to date. The resultant benefits would be numerous, including an increased inclination to invest in early years prevention, enhanced levels of confidence in VRUs on the part of partner agencies, and increased capacity for VRUs to work with one another to effect national-level policy change, including, for example, encouraging trauma-informed practice across a range of services working with children and young people.

Limitations and potential pitfalls

Before we conclude, it is important to acknowledge the limitations of the arguments presented in this book, along with the potential pitfalls associated with our analytical lens and the attendant implications for policy and practice.

Our focus has been on a particular form of violence: interpersonal violence committed by young people against their peers. Deciding on the scope of a research project and its outputs involves balancing breadth and depth. We chose to concentrate specifically on violence between young people in England and Wales due to the complexity of analysing different forms of violence that have distinct causes and are likely to require – to varying degrees – different responses. In addition, as recent policy initiatives associated with the public health approach to violence prevention in England and Wales have centred on preventing violence between young people, this necessarily inclined us towards a focus on this form of violence.

We would also argue, however, that many forms of violence share at least some common drivers. For instance, while shame and humiliation are recognised as key factors in making sense of violence between young people, studies suggest that they are also central to understanding honour-based violence (Welchman and Hossain, 2005), domestic violence (Dutton, 2006), and political violence (Stern, 2003). Moreover, the Four Is framework introduced and applied throughout this book is likely to prove useful for addressing these, and other, forms of violence. Preventing domestic violence, for instance, would benefit from action at the level of:

- societal inequalities (for example, addressing sexist norms, unequal access to employment opportunities, barriers to career progression, and the gender pay gap);
- institutions (for example, improving family and childhood support services);
- interventions (for example, the timely delivery of high-quality domestic violence perpetrator programmes);
- interactions (for example, foregrounding the importance of loving and healthy relationships between intimate partners in all of these levels).

These issues are complex and warrant further research and analysis beyond the scope of this book. Given the interconnections between different forms of violence, however, policy makers and practitioners would do well to avoid drawing overly rigid boundaries and distinctions when thinking about potential solutions to violence. During our interviews with VRU directors, a key debate emerged about whether VRUs should focus exclusively on violence between young people, or extend their scope to addressing other forms of violence, such as intimate partner violence and child abuse. Our perspective is that VRUs – and any organisation dedicated to safeguarding children and young people – should not limit their focus solely to violence occurring between young people and their peers. Due to their close connections, reducing violence perpetrated against children in the home, for instance, is likely to have positive spillover effects that help prevent violence later in life (Widom, 1989; Herrenkohl, 2008; Finkelhor et al, 2009).

In summary, while this book specifically addresses violence between young people, there appears to be significant overlap between the drivers of different forms of violence. We suggest that the Four Is framework for advancing the public health approach to violence prevention in England and Wales is likely to hold significant potential for addressing a much wider range of harmful behaviour beyond interpersonal violence committed by young people against other young people.

Conclusion

There is little harm more tragic and devastating than the loss of a young life, particularly when this loss comes at the hands of another young person. Among the most important features of any society are safe and secure environments for children and young people to flourish. Yet, in England and Wales today, far too many children and young people continue to be victims of serious violence and live in fear of violence. We can and must do better. To echo a phrase often promoted by the Scottish VRU (2020), 'violence is preventable, not inevitable'.

In recent years, a public health approach to violence prevention has emerged in England and Wales, the underpinning principles of which are endorsed in this book. However, putting principles into practice can be difficult. While our research has highlighted the tireless work of countless passionate and dedicated people and organisations, significant challenges remain. To address these challenges, we have provided a novel and comprehensive conceptual framework for the public health approach and argued why it offers a transformative path toward a low-violence society. To advance the public health approach to violence prevention in England and Wales, we propose adopting the Four Is framework, which calls for simultaneous action at four key levels: inequalities, institutions, interventions and interactions.

First, **inequalities**: Central governments must play their role in tackling a range of societal inequalities, including disparities in wealth, income, opportunity, recognition, and risk distribution.

Second, **institutions**: Societal institutions that shape the lives of children and young people, such as early childhood support services, schools, youth services, social work, health and mental health services, and youth justice, must be adequately resourced and work towards the pursuit of common and consistent goals.

Third, **interventions**: Effective interventions should be timely and targeted, ensuring the right support reaches the right individuals at the right times.

Finally, **interactions**: Consistent and high-quality interactions across a range of relationships in children and young people's lives – between peers, between parents and children, between teachers and students, between youth workers and young people, and so on – are crucial for preventing violence and fostering high levels of wellbeing, support, and safety.

Only through concerted action across all four of these levels can we achieve significant and sustained reductions in violence. This action must address the 'what', 'when', 'how', and 'where' of violence prevention:

- It must tackle the known determinants of violence operating at multiple levels, from the societal to the individual.
- It must operate at each stage of prevention (primary, secondary, and tertiary).
- It must consist of well-evaluated national and regional policies, and localised programmatic interventions.
- It must be driven by national, regional, and local-level governments and organisations.

Those who first articulated the public health approach to violence prevention envisioned an ambitious programme of action that extended well beyond the overreliance on multi-agency working initiatives and programmatic interventions that we see in present-day England and Wales. For the public health approach to violence prevention to fulfil its potential, we must return to these bold and ambitious visions, pursuing social and economic policies that reduce societal inequalities and enhance the quality of key institutions, infrastructure, and services that shape the quality of children and people's lives.

By doing so, this would significantly reduce the levels of shame, humiliation, and stigma experienced by many children and young people, and enhance young people's sense of mattering. This, as we have argued, is crucial to preventing much of the serious violence between young people that we see today. Only by taking concerted action along these lines will we be able to forge a path towards a peaceful society, where all children and young people can grow, thrive, flourish, and feel safe.

APPENDIX

Q-grid activity from VRU workshop

In September 2023, we invited all Violence Reduction Unit (VRU) directors in England, Scotland and Wales to a full-day, face-to-face workshop. The workshop covered a variety of topics, including key findings from the 'Public Health, Youth and Violence Reduction' (PHYVR) project, the implementation of the Serious Violence Duty, and engagement with young people and local communities. The final session of the day explored the issue of what a good VRU looks like and involved an activity that centred on the question: 'What criteria or achievements should VRUs be evaluated against?' A total of 46 people were split into six tables and asked to complete a 'Q-grid' that had been drawn on an A2 sheet on paper (see Figures A.1–A.6 later in this Appendix).

With its roots in the 1930s and a paper published in *Nature* by psychologist, William Stephenson (1935), Q Methodology has been used to good effect across a wide range of contexts and topics. Combining qualitative and quantitative approaches, it provides a systematic approach to exploring the subjective experiences and opinions of individuals and/or groups (Watts and Stenner, 2012).

The Q-grids provided to workshop participants consisted of nine columns, with the far-left column labelled 'least appropriate' and the far-right column labelled 'most appropriate'. The rows had no rank significance, but the further right a criteria/achievement was placed, the more it was felt appropriate as a way of evaluating the success of VRUs. Q-grids resemble inverted pyramids, with more options being placed in the central columns, and fewer towards the sides. In the context of the VRU workshop, the idea

Appendix

Figure A.1: Group A Q-grid

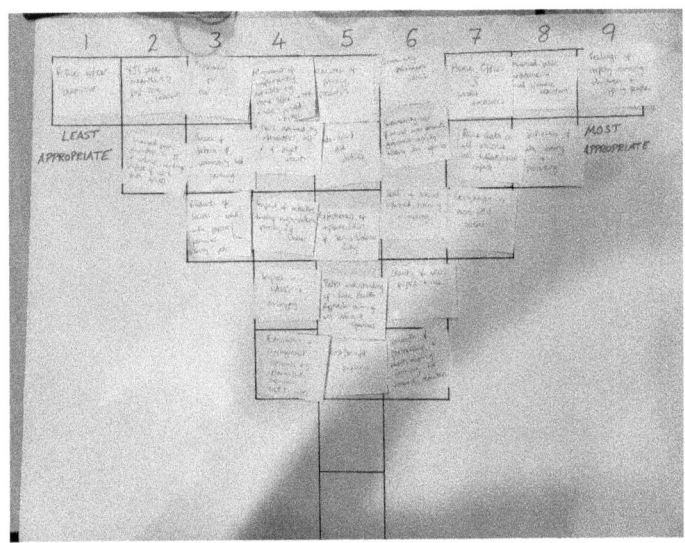

Figure A.2: Group B Q-grid

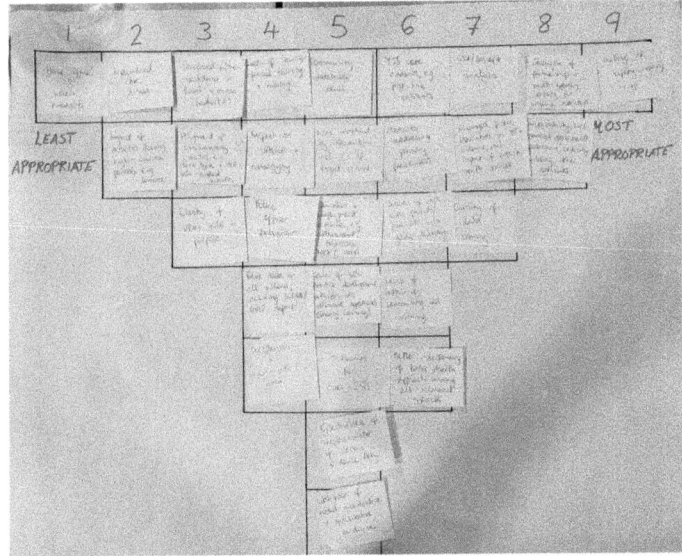

Figure A.3: Group C Q-grid

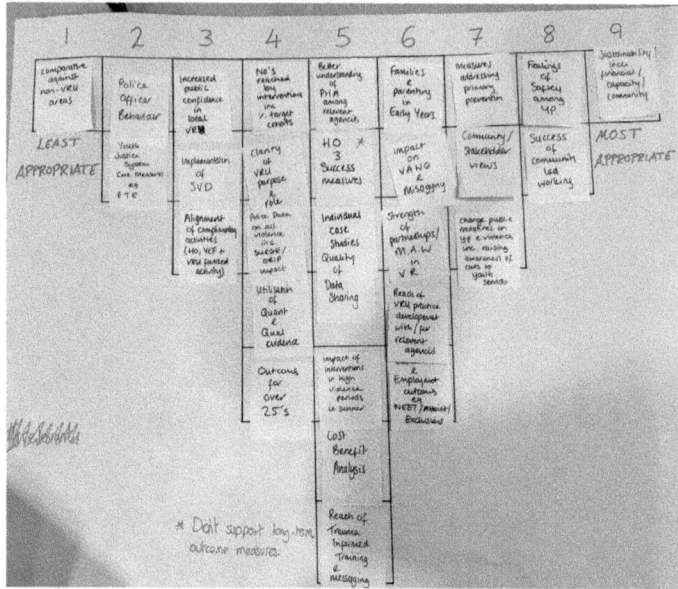

Figure A.4: Group D Q-grid

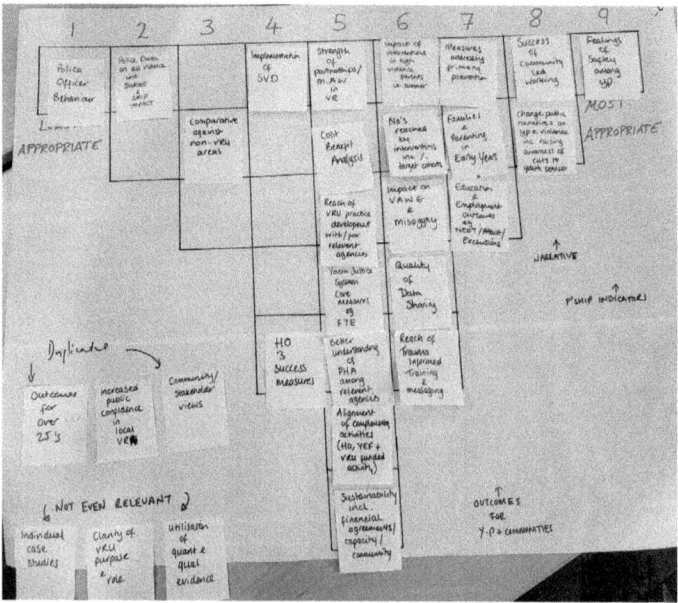

Appendix

Figure A.5: Group E Q-grid

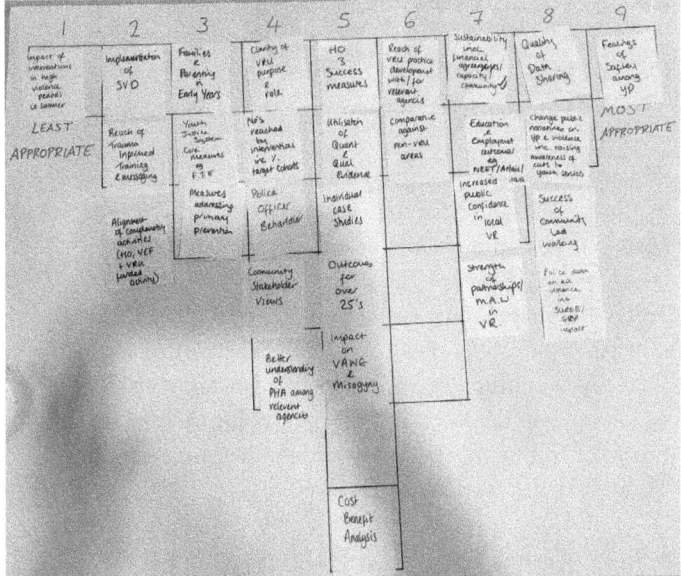

behind this activity was to encourage participants to identify what they saw as the most/least appropriate criteria/achievements, while stimulating debate and discussion as to their placement.

The criteria/achievements themselves had been created during the first session of the workshop, where participants had been asked to list all the possible criteria/achievements by which VRUs could possibly be evaluated. Two members of the PHYVR team then collated participants' responses and created sets of 29 possible criteria/achievements for use in the final session's Q-grid activity.

Each table spent around 40 minutes completing the Q-grids, before we went around the room summarising each table's grid and having a whole-group discussion based loosely on the following questions:

- What was your general rationale for the decisions you made?
- Have you found any criteria/achievements more difficult than others to sort? (Why was that?)

- Of the three criteria/achievements most important to you, why did you place them there and which is the most valuable to you?
- Of the three criteria/achievements least important to you, why did you place them there and which is the least valuable to you?
- How much consensus is there across each of the groups? What might the reasons be for this, and is consensus important, or not?
- How did you find the experience?

As noted in Chapter 5, none of the six groups placed either of the two primary outcome measures used in the annual Home Office evaluations – homicides and hospital admissions for injury by a sharp object – in the 'most appropriate' column. Instead, directors felt that the following criteria would be the most appropriate way of evaluating the success of VRUs:

- feelings of safety among children and young people (x4);
- sustainability (including financial, capacity, and community) (x1);
- success of community-led working (x1).

There were numerous reasons for directors' desires to downgrade the significance of the Home Office criteria, including the fact that they pushed VRUs towards tertiary violence reduction activities and a short-termist mindset. Any investment that VRUs made in primary prevention – for example, working to support families, parents, and carers with young children – would be unlikely to produce notable declines in homicides or hospital admissions in the coming months, and could therefore be seen as a wasted resource when viewed from the perspective of these relatively narrow metrics.

Instead, the vast majority of directors suggested that their work should be primarily aimed at enhancing feelings of safety and security among children and young people. This, so it was argued, would likely bring about reductions in serious violence by reducing levels of fear among young people that often sit at the heart of decisions – however misguided – to carry knives for protection (Nacro, 2023).

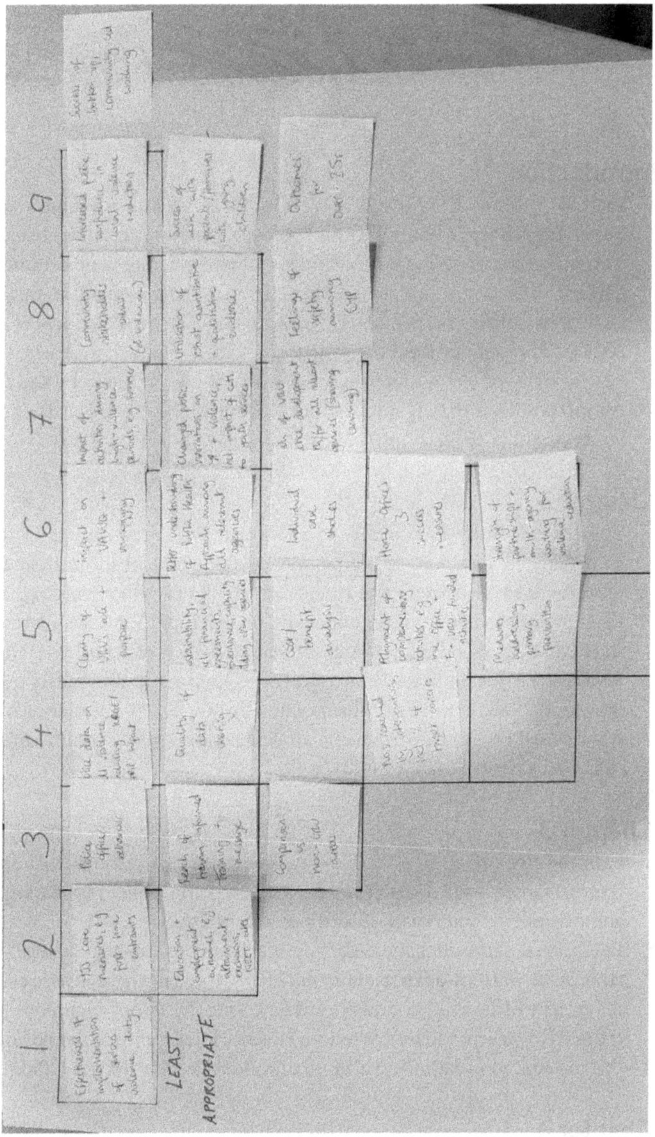

Appendix

Figure A.6: Group F Q-grid

Notes

Introduction
1. See ESRC Grant: ES/T005793/1, 'What Worked? Policy Mobility and the Public Health Approach to Youth Violence', www.changingviolence.org
2. The reason for using the term 'violence affecting young people' rather than 'violence affecting young men' is that girls and young women are frequently victims of violence perpetrated by young men (Office for National Statistics, 2024a). Throughout this book, the term is used with an awareness that the vast majority of serious interpersonal violence is committed by males.
3. All interviews are freely available for download via the UK Data Service, Study Number 9255: https://ukdataservice.ac.uk

Chapter 2
1. The term 'county lines' refers to the practice of urban gangs exploiting vulnerable children and young people, coercing and/or incentivising them to travel to smaller towns and rural areas to sell drugs (see Harding, 2020).
2. Keir Irwin-Rogers was lead criminologist on the Youth Violence Commission, and Irwin-Rogers and Luke Billingham were co-authors of its final report in 2020.
3. Similarly, a few months earlier, in response to a written parliamentary question in August 2018, Baroness Williams stated that the Serious Violence Strategy was focused on 'multi-partnership working and a "public health" approach' (UK Parliament, 2018).

Chapter 3
1. Community safety partnerships are multi-agency groups that include representatives from local services, including the police, probation, local authorities, fire and rescue authorities and health.
2. Educational authorities must comply with requests, so long as they: (i) are compatible with any other statutory duties; (ii) would not have adverse effects on the exercise of the education authority's functions; (iii) are not disproportionate to the need to prevent and reduce serious violence locally; and (iv) would not mean that the education authority incurred unreasonable costs (Home Office, 2022).

Chapter 4
1. The precise figure was 24 per cent, up from 19 per cent in the year ending March 2022, but down on the 32 per cent of preventative interventions in the year ending March 2021.

Notes

Chapter 5

1. This can apply whether or not one believes that people have 'free will' (see Harris, 2012).
2. Bellis et al (2017) have gone further to suggest that these levels should be extended beyond the national to the global, to take into account the interconnections between countries across the world, including, for example, international trade, migration, and shared planetary health issues such as global warming, all of which have serious implications for humanity as whole.
3. Two of this book's authors have published an accompanying policy briefing, which contains a more detailed list of policy and practice recommendations (see Irwin-Rogers and Billingham, 2024).

References

APPG Knife Crime (2019) *Back to School? Breaking the link between school exclusions and knife crime*, Barkingside: Barnardo's, Available from: https://www.barnardos.org.uk/sites/default/files/uploads/APPG%20on%20Knife%20Crime%20-%20Back%20to%20School_Breaking%20the%20links%20between%20school%20exclusions%20and%20knife%20crime%20October%202019.pdf [Accessed 22 November 2024].

Armstrong, D. (2004) 'A risky business? Research, policy, governmentality and youth offending', *Youth Justice*, 4(2): 100–16.

Arnez, J. and Condry, R. (2021) 'Criminological perspectives on school exclusion and youth offending', *Emotional and Behavioural Difficulties*, 26(1): 87–100.

Association of Police and Crime Commissioners (2023) 'PCCs making a difference: in focus: innovative and effective approaches to tackling serious violence', Available from: https://www.apccs.police.uk/campaigns/pccs-making-a-difference/ [Accessed 22 November 2024].

Atkinson, M., Wilkin, A., Stott, A., Doherty, P. and Kinder, K. (2002) 'Multi-agency working: a detailed study', National Foundation for Educational Research, Available from: https://www.nfer.ac.uk/publications/CSS02/CSS02.pdf [Accessed 22 November 2024].

Bannister, J., Bates, E. and Kearns, A. (2017) 'Local variance in the crime drop: a longitudinal study of neighbourhoods in greater Glasgow, Scotland', *The British Journal of Criminology*, 58(1): 177–99.

BBC News (2015) 'Scotland worst for violence – UN', BBC, Available from: http://news.bbc.co.uk/1/hi/scotland/4257966.stm [Accessed 22 November 2024].

References

Behavioural Insights Team (2020) 'Violence in London: what we know and how to respond', Available from: https://www.bi.team/wp-content/uploads/2020/02/BIT-London-Violence-Reduction.pdf [Accessed 22 November 2024].

Bellis, M., Hughes, K., Perkins, C. and Bennett, A. (2012) *Protecting People Promoting Health: A public health approach to violence prevention for England*, Department of Health, Available from: https://assets.publishing.service.gov.uk/government/uploads/system/uploads/attachment_data/file/216977/Violence-prevention.pdf [Accessed 22 November 2024].

Bellis, M., Hardcastle, K., Hughes, K., Wood, S. and Nurse, J. (2017) *Preventing Violence, Promoting Peace: A policy toolkit for preventing interpersonal, collective and extremist violence*, The Commonwealth Secretariat, Available from: https://phwwhocc.co.uk/wp-content/uploads/2020/08/Preventing-Violence-Promoting-Peace-Full-report.pdf [Accessed 22 November 2024].

Bellis, M., Hughes, K., Leckenby, N., Perkins, C. and Lowey, H. (2014) 'National household survey of adverse childhood experiences and their relationship with resilience to health-harming behaviours in England', *BMC*, 12(1): 72.

Big Lottery Fund (2018) Preventing Serious Youth Violence – What Works? Insights and Examples from the Community and Voluntary Sector', Available from: https://www.tnlcommunityfund.org.uk/media/documents/BLF_KL18-12-Serious-Violence.pdf [Accessed 27 January 2025].

Billingham, L. and Gillon, F. (2024) '(Re)moving exclusions: school exclusion reduction in Glasgow and London', *British Educational Research Journal*, 50(1): 287–306.

Billingham, L. and Irwin-Rogers, K. (2021) 'The terrifying abyss of insignificance: Marginalisation, mattering and violence between young people', *Oñati Socio-Legal Series*, 11(5): 1222–49.

Billingham, L. and Irwin-Rogers, K. (2022) *Against Youth Violence: A Social Harm Perspective*, Bristol: Bristol University Press.

Blagg, H. and Smith, D. (1989) *Crime, Penal Policy and Social Work*, Harlow: Pearson Longman.

Bottoms, A. and Dignan, J. (2004) 'Youth justice in Great Britain', *Crime and Justice: A Review of Research*, 31: 21–183.

Braga, A.A. and Weisburd, D. (2015) 'Focused deterrence and the prevention of violent gun injuries: practice, theoretical principles, and scientific evidence', *Annual Review of Public Health*, 36(1): 55–68.

Braga, A.A., Turchan, B. and Winship, C. (2019) 'Partnership, accountability, and innovation: Boston's experience with focused deterrence', in D. Weisburd and A.A. Braga (eds) *Police Innovation: Contrasting Perspectives*, Cambridge: Cambridge University Press.

Brewer, M., Fry, E. and Try, L. (2023) *The Living Standards Outlook 2023*, Available from: https://www.resolutionfoundation.org/app/uploads/2023/01/Living-Standards-Outlook-2023.pdf [Accessed 27 January 2025].

Bridges, L. (2021) 'The Police Bill, SVROs and guilt by association', Institute for Race Relations, Available from: https://irr.org.uk/article/police-bill-svros-guilt-by-association/ [Accessed 22 November 2024].

Brierley, A. (2021) *Connecting with Young People in Trouble*, Hook: Waterside Press.

Brown, D. (2018) 'Murder rate in London tops New York for the first time', *The Times*, 2 April 2018, Available from: https://www.thetimes.com/uk/article/murder-rate-in-london-tops-new-york-for-the-first-time-n78288ztb [Accessed 22 November 2024].

Brown, J. (2019) 'How is the government implementing a "public health approach" to serious violence?', Available from: https://commonslibrary.parliament.uk/how-is-the-government-implementing-a-public-health-approach-to-serious-violence/ [Accessed 22 November 2024].

Butts, J.A., Roman, C.G., Bostwick, L. and Porter, J.R. (2015) 'Cure violence: a public health model to reduce gun violence', *Annual Review of Public Health*, 36(1): 39–53.

Byrne, B., Alexander, C., Khan, O., Nazroo, J. and Shankley, W. (2020) (eds) *Ethnicity, Race and Inequality in the UK*, Bristol: Policy Press.

References

Cathro, C., Tagliaferri, G. and Sutherland, A. (2023) *School Exclusions and Youth Custody*, London: Behavioural Insights Team, Available from: https://www.bi.team/wp-content/uploads/2023/01/Nuffield-Foundation-Exclusions-and-Youth-Custody-Report-vFinal-2023-01-17.pdf [Accessed 22 November 2024].

Centers for Disease Control and Prevention (2017) *The Cardiff Violence Prevention Model Toolkit*, Atalanta: CDC.

Chaney, P. (2015) 'Popularism and punishment or rights and rehabilitation? Electoral discourse and structural policy narratives on youth justice: Westminster elections, 1964–2010', *Youth Justice*, 15(1): 23–41.

Child Poverty Action Group (2024a) 'Child poverty reaches record high – failure to tackle it will be 'a betrayal of Britain's children', Available from: https://cpag.org.uk/news/child-poverty-reaches-record-high-failure-tackle-it-will-be-betrayal-britains-children [Accessed 22 November 2024].

Child Poverty Action Group (2024b) 'Tackling child poverty: an urgent priority', Available from: https://cpag.org.uk/news/tackling-child-poverty-urgent-priority [Accessed 22 November 2024].

Children's Commissioner (2019) 'Exclusions: Children excluded from mainstream schools', Available from: https://assets.childrenscommissioner.gov.uk/wpuploads/2019/05/Exclusions-cover-merged.pdf [Accessed 27 January 2025].

Chonody, J., Ferman, B., Amitrani-Welsh, J. and Travis, M. (2013) 'Violence through the eyes of youth: a photovoice exploration', *Journal of Community Psychology*, 41(1): 84–101.

Cohen, D. (2018) 'Violent London: treat crimewave like public health emergency, experts say', *The Evening Standard*, 18 July 2018, Available from: https://www.standard.co.uk/news/crime/violent-london-treat-crimewave-like-public-health-emergency-experts-say-a3890321.html [Accessed 22 November 2024].

Coles, E., Cheyne, H., Rankin, J. and Daniel, B. (2016) 'Getting it Right for Every Child: a national policy framework to promote children's well-being in Scotland, United Kingdom', *Millbank Quarterly*, 94(2): 334–65.

Collins, R. (2008) *Violence: A micro-sociological theory*, Princeton, NJ: Princeton University Press.

Currie, E. (2016) *Roots of Danger: Violent crime in global perspective*, Oxford: Oxford University Press.

David-Ferdon, C., Vivolo-Kantor, A.M., Dahlberg, L.L., Marshall, K.J., Rainford, N. and Hall, J.E. (2016) *A Comprehensive Technical Package for the Prevention of Youth Violence and Associated Risk Behaviours*, National Center for Injury Prevention and Control, Available from: https://www.govinfo.gov/content/pkg/GOVPUB-HE20-PURL-gpo105863/pdf/GOVPUB-HE20-PURL-gpo105863.pdf [Accessed 27 January 2025].

Davidson, S. (1976) 'Planning and coordination of social services in multi-organisational contexts', *Social Services Review*, 50: 117–37.

Dawson, M.K., Ivey, A. and Buggs, S. (2023) 'Relationships, resources, and political empowerment: community violence intervention strategies that contest the logics of policing and incarceration', *Frontiers in Public Health*, 11: 1–7.

Department for Education (2024) 'School suspensions and permanent exclusion', Available from: https://www.gov.uk/government/publications/school-exclusion [Accessed 27 January 2025].

Department for Work and Pensions (2023) 'Households Below Average Income: an analysis of the UK income distribution: FYE 1995 to FYE 2022', Available from: https://www.gov.uk/government/statistics/households-below-average-income-for-financial-years-ending-1995-to-2022/households-below-average-income-an-analysis-of-the-uk-income-distribution-fye-1995-to-fye-2022 [Accessed 22 November 2024].

de St Croix, T. and Doherty, L. (2022) ' "Capturing the magic": grassroots perspectives on evaluating open youth work', *Journal of Youth Studies*, 27(4): 486–502.

Diamond, J. and Vangen, S. (2017) 'Coping with austerity: innovation via collaboration or retreat to the known', *Public Money & Management*, 37(1): 47–54.

Downes, D. and Newburn, T. (2022) *The Official History of Criminal Justice IV: The politics of law and order*, London: Routledge.

Drakeford, M. (2009) 'Children first, offenders second: youth justice in a devolved Wales', *Criminal Justice Matters*, no. 78, December.

References

Droste, N., Miller, P. and Baker, T. (2014) 'Emergency department data sharing to reduce alcohol-related violence: a systematic review of the feasibility and effectiveness of community-level interventions', *Emergency Medicine Australasia*, 26(4): 326–35.

Drury, I. (2017) 'Youth knife crime now at its highest level since 2009: courts deals with more than 4,400 cases involving 10 to 17-year-olds over 12-month period', *The Daily Mail*, 12 December 2017, Available from: https://www.dailymail.co.uk/news/article-5181517/Youth-knife-crime-highest-level-2009.html [Accessed 22 November 2024].

Dutton, D.G. (2006) *Rethinking Domestic Violence*, Vancouver: UBC Press.

Dwyer, P. and Micale, M. (2021) *The Darker Angels of Our Nature: Refuting the Pinker Theory of History and Violence*, New York: Bloomsbury Publishing.

Ellis, A. (2016) *Men, Masculinities and Violence*, London: Routledge.

Engel, R.S., Tillyer, M.S. and Corsaro, N. (2013) 'Reducing gang violence using focussed deterrence: evaluating the Cincinnati Initiative to Reduce Violence (CIRV)', *Justice Quarterly*, 30(3): 403–39.

Esmark, A. (2020) *The New Technocracy*, Bristol: Bristol University Press.

Evening Standard (2018) '*Evening Standard* comment: brutal night shows need for new plans on crime', Available from: https://www.standard.co.uk/comment/comment/evening-standard-comment-brutal-night-shows-need-for-new-plans-on-crime-a3902281.html [Accessed 22 November 2024].

Farrington, D.P. (2000) 'Explaining and preventing crime: the globalisation of knowledge: The American Society of Criminology 1999 Presidential Address', *Criminology*, 38(1): 1–24.

Farrington, D.P. (2005) 'Childhood origins of antisocial behavior', *Clinical Psychology and Psychotherapy*, 12(3): 177–90.

Finkelhor, D., Turner, H., Ormrod, R. and Hamby, S.L. (2009) 'Violence, abuse and crime exposure in a national sample of children and youth', *Pediatrics*, 124: 1411–23.

Firmin, C. (2020) *Contextual Safeguarding and Child Protection: Rewriting the rules*, London: Routledge.

Flett, G. (2018) *The Psychology of Mattering: Understanding the human need to be significant*, London: Academic Press.

Flyvbjerg, B. (2001) *Making Social Science Matter: Why social inquiry fails and how it can succeed again*, Cambridge: Cambridge University Press.

Fraser, A. (2017) *Gangs and Crime*, London: Sage.

Fraser, A. and Gillon, F. (2023) 'The Glasgow miracle? Storytelling, violence reduction and public policy', *Theoretical Criminology*, 28(3), DOI: 10.1177/13624806231208432.

Fraser, A. and Irwin-Rogers, K. (2021) 'A public health approach to violence reduction: Strategic Briefing 2021', Available from: https://www.researchinpractice.org.uk/all/publications/2021/july/a-public-health-approach-to-violence-reduction-strategic-briefing-2021/ [Accessed 22 November 2024].

Fraser, A., Billingham, L., Gillon, F., Irwin-Rogers, K., McVie, S. and Newburn, T. (forthcoming) *A Public Health Approach to Violence Reduction*, Oxford: Oxford University Press.

Fraser, A., Irwin-Rogers, K., Gillon, F., Billingham, L., McVie, S. and Schwarze, T. (2024) *Safe Space: The past and present of violence reduction in Scotland*, Glasgow: SCCJR, Available from: https://www.sccjr.ac.uk/publication/safe-space-the-past-present-future-of-violence-reduction-in-scotland/ [Accessed 22 November 2024].

Garland, D. (1985) *Punishment and Welfare: A history of penal strategies*, Aldershot: Gower.

Gilligan, J. (1996) *Violence: Reflections on a national epidemic*, New York, NY: Vintage Books.

Gilligan, J. (2001) *Preventing Violence*, New York, NY: Thames & Hudson.

Goddard, T. (2014) 'The indeterminacy of the risk factor prevention paradigm: a case study of community partnerships implementing youth and gang violence prevention policy', *Youth Justice*, 14(1): 3–21.

Goldson, B. (2020) 'Excavating youth justice reform: historical mapping and speculative prospects', *The Howard Journal of Crime and Justice*, 59(3): 317–34.

Gourtsoyannis, P. (2019) 'Theresa May hails Scotland's approach on knife crime', *The Scotsman*, 6 March 2019, Available from: https://www.scotsman.com/news/politics/theresa-may-hails-scotlands-approach-on-knife-crime-87996 [Accessed 22 November 2024].

References

Gray, P., Jump, D. and Smithson, H. (2023) *Adverse Childhood Experiences and Serious Youth Violence*, Bristol: Bristol University Press.

Grimshaw, R. and Ford, M. (2018) *Young People, Violence and Knives: Revisiting the evidence and policy discussions*, London: Centre for Crime and Justice Studies.

The Guardian (2005) 'Corrections and clarifications', 24 October, Available from: https://www.theguardian.com/news/2005/oct/24/mainsection.correctionsandclarifications [Accessed 13 January 2025].

Haines, K. (2009) 'The dragonisation of youth justice', in W. Taylor, R. Earle and R. Hester (eds) *Youth Justice Handbook: Theory, policy and practice*, Cullompton: Willan.

Hansard (2018) 'Public health model to reduce youth violence', volume 651, Available from: https://hansard.parliament.uk/commons/2018-12-13/debates/2DAF6086-57A3-492E-8AB4-DDC207EAA03D/PublicHealthModelToReduceYouthViolence [Accessed 22 November 2024].

Hansard (2023) 'Stop and search', volume 734, Available from: https://hansard.parliament.uk/Commons/2023-06-19/debates/B7DE2421-85FA-432D-967E-57FE8F5240D8/StopAndSearch [Accessed 22 November 2024].

Hansard (2024) 'Knife crime: Violence Reduction Units', volume 836, Available from: https://hansard.parliament.uk/Lords/2024-02-20/debates/DF586CEE-7DDB-42EE-842C-CED3EE8BE721/KnifeCrimeViolenceReductionUnits [Accessed 22 November 2024].

Harding, S. (2014) *The Street Casino: Survival in violence street gangs*, Bristol: Bristol University Press.

Harding, S. (2020) *County Lines: Exploitation and drug dealing among urban street gangs*, Bristol: Bristol University Press.

Harris, R. (1982) 'Institutionalised ambivalence: social work and the Children and Young Persons Act *1969*', *The British Journal of Social Work*, 12(3): 247–63.

Harris, S. (2012) *Free Will*, New York, NY: Free Press.

The Health Foundation (2024) 'Trends in people needing emergency temporary accommodation', Available from: https://www.health.org.uk/evidence-hub/housing/housing-stability-and-security/trends-in-people-needing-emergency-temporary [Accessed 27 January 2025].

Henley, J. (2011) 'Karyn McCluskey: the woman who took on Glasgow's gangs', *The Guardian*, 19 December 2011, Available from: https://www.theguardian.com/society/2011/dec/19/karyn-mccluskey-glasgow-gangs [Accessed 22 November 2024].

Herrenkohl, T.I., Sousa, C., Tajima, E.A., Herrenkohl, R.C. and Moylan, C.A. (2008) 'Intersection of child abuse and children's exposure to domestic violence', *Trauma, Violence and Abuse*, 9(2): 84–99.

Hill, M., Walker, M., Moodie, K., Wallace, B., Bannister, J., Khan, F., McIvor, G. and Kendrick, A. (2005) *Fast Track Children's Hearings Pilot: Final report of the evaluation of a pilot*, Edinburgh: National Records of Scotland, Available from: https://webarchive.nrscotland.gov.uk/20201121213732/http://www2.gov.scot/Publications/2005/06/14103237/32402 [Accessed 22 November 2024].

His Majesty's Inspectorate of Constabulary and Fire & Rescue Services (2023) 'An inspection of how well the police tackle serious youth violence', Available from: https://hmicfrs.justiceinspectorates.gov.uk/publication-html/inspection-of-how-well-the-police-tackle-serious-youth-violence/#implementing-a-public-health-approach [Accessed 22 November 2024].

HM Government (2011) *Ending Gang and Youth Violence: A cross-government report*, Cm. 8211, London: The Stationery Office.

HMIP (2023) *Children in Custody 2022–23*, Available from: https://www.justiceinspectorates.gov.uk/hmiprisons/wp-content/uploads/sites/4/2023/11/Children-in-custody-web-2023-2.pdf [Accessed 27 January 2025].

HM Prison and Probation Service (2024) 'Youth custody data', Available from: https://www.gov.uk/government/publications/youth-custody-data [Accessed 22 November 2024].

Hock, E.S., Blank, L., Fairbrother, H., Clowes, M., Cuevas, D.C., Booth, A., Clair, A. and Goyder, E. (2024) 'Exploring the impact of housing insecurity on the health and wellbeing of children and young people in the United Kingdom: a qualitative systematic review', *BMC Public Health*, 24: 2453.

References

Home Affairs Committee (2019) ' "Youth Service Guarantee" needed to protect young people from serious violence', Available from: https://committees.parliament.uk/work/3152/serious-violence-inquiry/news/100498/youth-service-guarantee-needed-to-protect-young-people-from-serious-violence/ [Accessed 22 November 2024].

Home Office (1965) *The Child, the Family and the Young Offender*, Cmnd 2742, London: Her Majesty's Stationery Office.

Home Office (2018a) 'Home Office hosts first serious violence event in London', Available from: https://www.gov.uk/government/news/home-office-hosts-first-serious-violence-event-in-london [Accessed 22 November 2024].

Home Office (2018b) 'Serious Violence Strategy', Available from: https://assets.publishing.service.gov.uk/government/uploads/system/uploads/attachment_data/file/698009/serious-violence-strategy.pdf [Accessed 22 November 2024].

Home Office (2018c) 'Youth Endowment Fund: advert', Available from: https://www.gov.uk/government/publications/youth-endowment-fund-call-for-proposals [Accessed 22 November 2024].

Home Office (2018d) 'Youth Endowment Fund: prospectus', Available from: https://www.gov.uk/government/publications/youth-endowment-fund-call-for-proposals [Accessed 22 November 2024].

Home Office (2018e) 'Home Secretary launches Serious Violence Strategy', press release, Available from: https://www.gov.uk/government/news/home-secretary-to-launch-serious-violence-strategy [Accessed 27 January 2025].

Home Office (2019a) 'Charity chosen to deliver £200m Youth Endowment Fund to tackle violence', Available from: https://www.gov.uk/government/news/charity-chosen-to-deliver-200m-youth-endowment-fund-to-tackle-violence [Accessed 22 November 2024].

Home Office (2019b) 'Consultation on a new legal duty to support a multi-agency approach to preventing and tackling serious violence: government response', Available from: https://assets.publishing.service.gov.uk/government/uploads/system/uploads/attachment_data/file/816885/Government_Response_-_Serious_Violence_Consultation_Final.pdf [Accessed 22 November 2024].

Home Office (2019c) 'Funding for Violence Reduction Units announced', Available from: https://www.gov.uk/government/news/funding-for-violence-reduction-units-announced [Accessed 22 November 2024].

Home Office (2019d) 'What is the government doing to tackle violent crime?', Available from: https://homeofficemedia.blog.gov.uk/2019/06/18/what-is-the-government-doing-to-tackle-violent-crime-2/ [Accessed 22 November 2024].

Home Office (2019e) 'New public health duty to tackle serious violence', Available from: https://www.gov.uk/government/news/new-public-health-duty-to-tackle-serious-violence [Accessed 22 November 2024].

Home Office (2019f) 'Consultation on a new legal duty to support a multi-agency approach to preventing and tackling serious violence', Available from: https://assets.publishing.service.gov.uk/government/uploads/system/uploads/attachment_data/file/816885/Government_Response_-_Serious_Violence_Consultation_Final.pdf [Accessed 22 November 2024].

Home Office (2019g) 'Preventing serious violence: summary', Available from: https://www.gov.uk/government/publications/preventing-serious-violence-a-multi-agency-approach/preventing-serious-violence-summary#:~:text=A%20new%20legal%20duty%20to,to%20the%20Youth%20Endowment%20Fund [Accessed 22 November 2024].

Home Office (2019h) 'Serious youth violence summit to launch public health duty to tackle serious violence', Available from: https://www.gov.uk/government/news/serious-youth-violence-summit-to-launch-public-health-duty-to-tackle-serious-violence [Accessed 22 November 2024].

References

Home Office (2019i) 'Home Office allocates £35 million to police forces for violence reduction units', Available from: https://www.gov.uk/government/news/home-office-allocates-35-million-to-police-forces-for-violence-reduction-units#:~:text=Home%20Secretary%20Sajid%20Javid%20said,to%20stop%20this%20senseless%20bloodshed [Accessed 27 January 2025].

Home Office (2020a) 'Process evaluation of the Violence Reduction Units', Available from: https://assets.publishing.service.gov.uk/government/uploads/system/uploads/attachment_data/file/910822/process-evaluation-of-the-violence-reduction-units-horr116.pdf [Accessed 22 November 2024].

Home Office (2020b) 'Violence Reduction Unit interim guidance', Available from: https://assets.publishing.service.gov.uk/government/uploads/system/uploads/attachment_data/file/876380/12VRU_Interim_Guidance_FINAL__003_2732020.pdf [Accessed 22 November 2024].

Home Office (2021) 'Knife Crime Prevention Orders', Available from: https://assets.publishing.service.gov.uk/government/uploads/system/uploads/attachment_data/file/1052327/KCPO_Framework_Guidance_-_July_2021_-_FINAL-SENT-APPROVED-FOR_PUBLICATION_-_REVIEWED_JAN_2022.pdf [Accessed 22 November 2024].

Home Office (2022a) 'Serious Violence Duty statutory guidance', Available from: https://assets.publishing.service.gov.uk/government/uploads/system/uploads/attachment_data/file/1125001/Final_Serious_Violence_Duty_Statutory_Guidance_-_December_2022.pdf [Accessed 22 November 2024].

Home Office (2022b) 'Home Secretary backs police to increase stop and search', Available from: https://www.gov.uk/government/news/home-secretary-backs-police-to-increase-stop-and-search [Accessed 22 November 2024].

Home Office (2022c) 'Violence reduction unit year ending March 2021 evaluation report', Available from: https://www.gov.uk/government/publications/violence-reduction-unit-year-ending-march-2021-evaluation-report [Accessed 27 January 2025].

Home Office (2023a) 'Police urged to use stop and search to save more lives', Available from: https://www.gov.uk/government/news/police-urged-to-use-stop-and-search-to-save-more-lives [Accessed 22 November 2024].

Home Office (2023b) 'Serious violence: funding allocations', Available from: https://www.gov.uk/government/publications/serious-violence-funding-allocations/serious-violence-funding-allocations [Accessed 22 November 2024].

Home Office (2023c) 'Violence Reduction Units 2022 to 2023', Available from: https://www.gov.uk/government/publications/violence-reduction-units-year-ending-march-2023-evaluation-report/violence-reduction-units-2022-to-2023 [Accessed 22 November 2024].

Home Office (2023d) 'Violence Reduction Units, year ending March 2022 evaluation report', Available from: https://www.gov.uk/government/publications/violence-reduction-units-year-ending-march-2022-evaluation-report [Accessed 27 January 2025].

Hood, R., Goldacre, A., Gorin, S. and Bywaters, P. (2020) 'Screen, ration and churn: demand management and the crisis in children's social care', *British Journal of Social Work*, 50: 868–89.

Hood, R., Price, J., Sartori, D., Maisey, D., Johnson, J. and Clark, Z. (2017) 'Collaborating across the threshold: the development of interprofessional expertise in child safeguarding', *Journal of Interprofessional Care*, 31(6): 705–13.

Hope Collective (2022a) 'About the Hope Collective', Available from: https://www.hopecollectiveuk.org/ [Accessed 22 November 2024].

Hope Collective (2022b) 'Changing the conversation', Available from: https://static1.squarespace.com/static/627e1c0abbf4f73ea393f0e0/t/62b9ecec1814b4697b607c0d/1656351989648/Hope-Collective-Changing-The-Conversation.pdf [Accessed 22 November 2024].

Horwath, J. and Morrison, T. (2007) 'Collaboration, integration and change in children's services: critical issues and key ingredients', *Child Abuse & Neglect*, 31: 55–69.

Hothersall, S.J. (2012) *Social Work with Children, Young People and their Families in Scotland*, London: Learning Matters.

House of Commons Library (2019) 'How is the government implementing a "public health approach" to serious violence?', Available from: https://commonslibrary.parliament.uk/how-is-the-government-implementing-a-public-health-approach-to-serious-violence/ [Accessed 22 November 2024].

References

House of Commons Library (2023) 'Knife crime in England & Wales: statistics', Available from: https://researchbriefings.files.parliament.uk/documents/SN04304/SN04304.pdf [Accessed 22 November 2024].

Hurtubise, K. and Joslin, R. (2023) 'Participant-generated timelines: a participatory tool to explore young people with chronic pain and parents' narratives of their healthcare experiences', *Qualitative Health Research*, 33(11): 931–44.

Hymans, M. (2008) 'How personal constructs about "professional identity" might act as a barrier to multi-agency working', *Educational Psychology in Practice*, 24(4): 279–88.

Irwin-Rogers, K. (2019) 'Illicit drug markets, consumer capitalism and the rise of social media: a toxic trap for young people', *Critical Criminology*, 27: 591–610.

Irwin-Rogers, K. and Billingham, L. (2024) 'A safer society for young people: advancing a public health approach to violence prevention', Available from: https://changingviolence.org/publications/a-safer-society-for-young-people-advancing-a-public-health-approach-to-violence-prevention/ [Accessed 22 November 2024].

Irwin-Rogers, K., Muthoo, A. and Billingham, L. (2020) *Youth Violence Commission: Final report*, Youth Violence Commission, Available from: https://www.yvcommission.com [Accessed 22 November 2024].

Jabar, A., Fong, F., Chavira, M., Cerqueira, M.T., Barth, D., Matzopoulos, R. and Engel, M.E. (2019) 'Is the introduction of violence and injury observatories associated with a reduction in violence-related injury in adult populations? A systematic review and meta-analysis', *BMJ Open*, 9(7): e027977.

Jerrim, J., Sims, S. and Taylor, H. (2021) 'I quit! Is there an association between leaving teaching and improvements in mental health?', *British Educational Research Journal*, 47(3): 692–724.

Johnstone, G. and Bottomley, K. (1998) 'Introduction: Labour's crime policy in context', *Policy Studies*, 19(3–4): 173–84.

Jones, G., Jackson, T., Ahmed, H., Brown, Q., Dantzler, T., Ford, N. et al (2021) 'Youth voices in violence prevention', *American Journal of Public Health*, 111: 17–19.

Jones, R. and Whitehead, M. (2018) '"Politics done like science": Critical perspectives on psychological governance and the experimental state', *Environment and Planning D: Society and Space*, 36(2): 313–30.

Joseph Rowntree Foundation (2023) 'Deep poverty and destitution', Available from: https://www.jrf.org.uk/deep-poverty-and-destitution [Accessed 27 January 2025].

Junger-Tas, J. (2006) 'Trends in international juvenile justice; what conclusions can be drawn?', in J. Junger-Tas and S. Decker (eds) *International Handbook of Juvenile Justice*, Dordrecht: Springer.

Kennedy, D.M. (2006) 'Old wine in new bottles: policing and the lessons of pulling levers', in D. Weisburd and A.A. Braga (eds) *Police Innovation: Contrasting Perspectives*, Cambridge: Cambridge University Press: 155–70.

Kennedy, D.M. (2019) 'Policing and the lessons of focused deterrence', in D. Weisburd and A.A. Braga (eds) *Police Innovation: Contrasting perspectives*, Cambridge: Cambridge University Press.

Kennedy, D.M., Braga, A.A., Piehl, A.M. and Waring, E.J. (2001) *Reducing Gun Violence: The Boston Gun Project's Operation Ceasefire*, Washington DC: U.S. Department of Justice.

Krug, E.G., Dahlberg, L.L., Mercy, J.A., Zwi, A.B. and Lozano, R. (2002) *World Report on Violence and Health*, Geneva: World Health Organization, Available from: https://apps.who.int/iris/bitstream/handle/10665/42495/9241545615_eng.pdf [Accessed 22 November 2024].

Labour (1997) *New Labour because Britain deserves better*, 1997 Labour Party Manifesto, Available from: http://www.labour-party.org.uk/manifestos/1997/1997-labour-manifesto.shtml [Accessed 13 January 2025].

Labour (2023) 'Labour announces new "tough love" youth programme to tackle knife crime, youth violence and address the crisis in young people's mental health', Available from: https://labour.org.uk/updates/press-releases/labour-announces-new-tough-love-youth-programme-to-tackle-knife-crime-youth-violence-and-address-the-crisis-in-young-peoples-mental-health/ [Accessed 22 November 2024].

References

Labour (2024) 'Mission-driven government', Available from: https://labour.org.uk/change/mission-driven-government/ [Accessed 22 November 2024].

Layder, D. (1998) *Sociological Practice: Linking theory and social research*, London: Sage.

Lightowler, C., Orr, D. and Vaswani, N. (2014) *Youth Justice in Scotland: Fixed in the past or fit for the future*, Strathclyde: Centre for Youth and Criminal Justice, Available from: http://www.cycj.org.uk/wp-content/uploads/2014/09/Youth-Justice-in-Scotland.pdf [Accessed 22 November 2024].

Loebach, J., Little, S., Cox, A. and Owens, P.E. (eds) *The Routledge Handbook of Designing Public Spaces for Young People: Processes, practices and policies for youth inclusion*, London: Routledge.

Loeber, R. and Stouthamer-Loeber, M. (1998) 'Development of juvenile aggression and violence: some common misconceptions and controversies', *American Psychologist*, 53(2): 242–59.

London Violence Reduction Unit (2024) 'London's Inclusion Charter', Available from: https://www.london.gov.uk/programmes/communities-and-social-justice/londons-violence-reduction-unit-vru/londons-inclusion-charter [Accessed 22 November 2024].

Ludwig, J., Duncan, G.J. and Hirschfield, P. (2001) 'Urban poverty and juvenile crime: Evidence from a randomized housing-mobility experiment', *Quarterly Journal of Economics*, 116(2): 655–79.

Luguetti, C., Ryan, J., Eckersley, B., Howard, A., Buck, S., Osman, A. et al (2024) '"It wasn't adults and young people […] we're all in it together": co-designing a post-secondary transition program through youth participatory action research', *Education Action Research*, 32(4): 641–58.

Manzoni, J. (2017) 'Big data in government: the challenges and opportunities', Available from: https://www.gov.uk/government/speeches/big-data-in-government-the-challenges-and-opportunities [Accessed 22 November 2024].

May, T. and Javid, S. (2019) 'We need a new way to treat the sickness of knife violence, write Theresa May and Sajid Javid', *Mail Online*, 31 March 2019, Available from: https://www.dailymail.co.uk/debate/article-6870873/We-need-new-way-treat-sickness-knife-violence-write-THERESA-SAJID-JAVID.html [Accessed 22 November 2024].

Mayor of Greater Manchester (2023) [Twitter] 23 August, Available from: https://x.com/MayorofGM/status/1694346190408610059 [Accessed 22 November 2024].

Mayor of London (2018) 'Mayor launches new public health approach to tackling serious violence', Available from: https://www.london.gov.uk/press-releases/mayoral/new-public-health-approach-to-tackling-violence [Accessed 22 November 2024].

Mayor of London (2022) 'The Violence Reduction Unit (VRU) 2022–2023 Funding Programme', Available from: https://www.london.gov.uk/programmes-strategies/mayors-office-policing-and-crime/governance-and-decision-making/mopac-decisions-0/violence-reduction-unit-vru-2022-2023-funding-programme [Accessed 22 November 2024].

McAra, L. (2006) 'Welfare in crisis? Youth justice in Scotland', in J. Muncie and B. Goldson (eds) *Comparative Youth Justice*, London: Sage.

McAra, L. (2010) 'Scottish youth justice: convergent pressures and cultural singularities', in F. Bailleau and Y. Cartuyvels (eds) *The Criminalisation of Youth: Juvenile justice in Europe, Turkey and Canada*, Brussels: VUB Press.

McAra, L. (2017) 'Youth justice', in A. Liebling, L. McAra and S. Maruna (eds) *Oxford Handbook of Criminology*, 6th ed., Oxford: Oxford University Press: 938–66.

McAra, L. and McVie, S. (2010) 'Youth justice in Scotland', in H. Croall, G. Mooney and M. Munro (eds) *Criminal Justice in Scotland*, Cullompton: Willan.

McAra, L. and McVie, S. (2013) 'Delivering justice for children and young people: Key messages from the Edinburgh Study of Youth Transitions and Crime', in *Justice for Young People: Papers by Winners of the Research Medal 2013*, pp 3–14.

McAra, L. and McVie, S. (2018) 'Transformations in youth crime and justice across Europe: evidencing the case for diversion', in B. Goldson (ed) *Juvenile Justice in Europe: Past, present and future*, London: Routledge.

McAra, L. and McVie, S. (2024) 'A quiet revolution: what worked to create a "whole system approach" to juvenile justice in Scotland', in C.M. Langton and J.R. Worling (eds) *What Works With Adolescents Who Have Offended: Theory, research, and practice*, Hoboken, NJ: Wiley Blackwell.

McLean, R. (2019) *Gangs, Drugs and (Dis)Organised Crime*, Bristol: Bristol University Press.

McNeill, F. and Batchelor, S. (2004) 'Persistent offending by young people: developing practice', *Issues in Community and Criminal Justice*, (3), London: National Association of Probation Officers.

McVie, S. (2017) 'Social order: crime and justice in Scotland', in D. McCrone (ed) *The New Sociology of Scotland*, London: Sage: 293–322.

McVie, S., Bates, E. and Pillinger, R. (2018) 'Changing patterns of violence in Glasgow and London: is there evidence of Scottish exceptionalism?', Available from: https://blogs.lse.ac.uk/politicsandpolicy/patterns-of-violence-glasgow-london/ [Accessed 22 November 2024].

McVie, S., Norris, P. and Pillinger, R. (2020) 'Increasing inequality in experience of victimisation during the crime drop: analysing patterns of victimisation in Scotland from 1993 to 2014–15', *British Journal of Criminology*, 60(3): 782–802.

Messner, S.F. and Rosenfeld, R. (2013) *Crime and the Economy*, Los Angeles: Sage.

Ministry of Housing, Communities and Local Government (2024) 'Statutory homelessness in England: financial year 2023–24', Available from: https://www.gov.uk/government/statistics/statutory-homelessness-in-england-financial-year-2023-24/statutory-homelessness-in-england-financial-year-2023-24 [Accessed 27 January 2025].

Molloy, M. (2018) 'London stabbings: 300 extra police deployed on streets to tackle spike in knife crime', Available from: https://www.telegraph.co.uk/news/2018/04/07/london-stabbings-300-extra-police-deployed-streets-tackle-spike/ [Accessed 22 November 2024].

Morenoff, J.D., Sampson, R.J. and Raudenbush, S.W. (2001) 'Neighborhood Inequality, Collective Efficacy, and the Spatial Dynamics of Urban Violence', Criminology, 39(3): 517–58.

Morgan, R. and Newburn, T. (2007) 'Youth justice', in M. Maguire, R. Morgan and R. Reiner (eds) *Oxford Handbook of Criminology*, 4th ed, Oxford: Oxford University Press.

Metropolitan Police Service (2021) 'Met Crime Data Dashboard', Available from: www.met.police.uk/sd/stats-and-data/met/homicide-dashboard/ [Accessed 22 November 2024].

Nacro (2023) *Lives not Knives: Young people's perspectives on knife crime*, London: Nacro, Available from: https://www.nacro.org.uk/wp-content/uploads/2023/01/Lives-Not-Knives_-young-peoples-perspective-on-knife-crime.pdf [Accessed 22 November 2024].

National Youth Agency (2024) *National Youth Sector Census: Snapshot, Summer 2024*, Leicester: NYA, Available from: https://nya.org.uk/wp-content/uploads/2024/09/1712-NYA-Census-Snapshot-Report_P3_DIGITAL.pdf [Accessed 22 November 2024].

Newburn, T., Deacon, R., Diski, R., Cooper, K., Grant, M. and Burch, A. (2016a) '"The best three days of my life": pleasure, power and alienation in the 2011 riots', *Crime, Media, Culture*, 14(1): 41–59.

Newburn, T., Diski, R., Cooper, K., Deacon, R., Burch, A. and Grant, M. (2016b) '"The biggest gang": police and people in the 2011 England riots', *Policing and Society*, 28(2): 205–22.

NHS Digital (2023) 'Hospital admitted patient care activity, 2022–23', Available from: https://digital.nhs.uk/data-and-information/publications/statistical/hospital-admitted-patient-care-activity/2022-23 [Accessed 22 November 2024].

Norberg, J. (2016) *Progress: Ten reasons to look forward to the future*, London: Oneworld Publications.

Norris, N. and Kushner, S. (2007) 'The New Public Management and evaluation', in S. Kushner and N. Norris (eds) *Dilemmas of Engagement: Evaluation and the New Public Management (Advances in Program Evaluation, Vol. 10)*, Bingley: Emerald Group Publishing Limited: 1–16.

References

Office for National Statistics (2017) 'Public perceptions of crime in England and Wales: year ending March 2016', Available from: https://www.ons.gov.uk/peoplepopulationandcommunity/crimeandjustice/articles/publicperceptionsofcrimeinenglandandwales/yearendingmarch2016#worry-about-crime [Accessed 22 November 2024].

Office for National Statistics (2023) 'Crime Survey for England and Wales: year ending June 2023', Available from: https://www.ons.gov.uk/peoplepopulationandcommunity/crimeandjustice/bulletins/crimeinenglandandwales/yearendingjune2023#:~:text=6.-,Violence,the%20year%20ending%20June%202022 [Accessed 22 November 2024].

Office for National Statistics (2024a) 'Crime in England and Wales: year ending December 2023', Available from: https://www.ons.gov.uk/peoplepopulationandcommunity/crimeandjustice/bulletins/crimeinenglandandwales/yearendingdecember2023#violence [Accessed 22 November 2024].

Office for National Statistics (2024b) 'Homicide in England and Wales: year ending March 2023', Available from: https://www.ons.gov.uk/peoplepopulationandcommunity/crimeandjustice/articles/homicideinenglandandwales/yearendingmarch2023 [Accessed 22 November 2024].

Office for National Statistics (2024c) 'Young people not in eduction, employment or training (NEET), UK: November 2024', Available from: https://www.ons.gov.uk/employmentandlabourmarket/peoplenotinwork/unemployment/bulletins/youngpeoplenotineducationemploymentortrainingneet/november2024 [Accessed 27 January 2025].

Organisation for Economic Co-operation and Development (2024) 'Income inequality dataset', Available from: https://data.oecd.org/inequality/income-inequality.htm [Accessed 22 November 2024].

Owens, R. and Lloyd, J. (2023) 'From behaviour-based to ecological: multi-agency partnership responses to extra-familial harm', *Journal of Social Work*, 23(4): 741–60.

Pardini, D.A., Raine, A., Erickon, K. and Loeber, R. (2014) 'Lower amygdala volume in men is associated with childhood aggression, early psychopathic traits, and future violence', *Biological Psychiatry*, 75(1): 73–80.

Pardo-Beneyto, G. and Abellan-Lopez, M.A. (2023) 'Participatory budgeting for young people as democratic socialisation: an approach to the case of Spain', *Children and Society*, 37(5): 1555–75.

Peters, B.G. (2017) 'What is so wicked about wicked problems? A conceptual analysis and a research program', *Policy and Society*, 36(3): 385–96.

Piketty, T. (2020) *Capital and Ideology*, Cambridge, MA: Harvard University Press.

Pinker, S. (2011) *The Better Angels of our Nature*, New York, NY: Viking Penguin.

Pinker, S. (2018) *Enlightenment Now: The case for reason, science, humanism and progress*, New York, NY: Penguin.

Pollitt, C. (2001) 'Convergence: the useful myth?', *Public Administration*, 79(4): 933–47.

Prison Reform Trust (2021) *Bromley Briefings Prison Factfile: Winter 2021*, Available from: https://prisonreformtrust.org.uk/wp-content/uploads/2022/01/Bromley_Briefings_winter_2021.pdf [Accessed 27 January 2025].

Public Health England (2019) 'A whole-system multi-agency approach to serious violence prevention', Available from: https://assets.publishing.service.gov.uk/media/5e38133d40f0b609169cb532/multi-agency_approach_to_serious_violence_prevention.pdf [Accessed 22 November 2024].

Raine, A. (2013) *The Anatomy of Violence: The biological roots of crime*, London: Penguin Group.

Raine, A. (2019) 'A neurodevelopmental perspective on male violence', *Infant Mental Health Journal*, 40(1): 84–97.

Ravalier, J., Wainwright, E., Clabburn, O., Loon, M. and Smyth, N. (2021) 'Working conditions and wellbeing in UK social workers', *Journal of Social Work*, 21(5): 1105–23.

Reich, R.B. (2016) *Saving Capitalism: For the many, not the few*, New York, NY: Vintage Books.

Rennie, N. (2024) *Violence Reduction Units at a Crossroads: The potential road ahead?*, Ayr: New Routes Consulting.

Richardson, H. (2023) 'Professional identity as a barrier to inter-agency working? A meta-ethnography of research conducted with professionals working with UK children's services', *Journal of Children's Services*, 18(2): 104–20.

References

Ridley, M. (2011) *The Rational Optimist: How prosperity evolves*, New York, NY: HarperCollins.

Riemann, M. (2019) 'Problematising the medicalization of violence: a critical discourse analysis of the 'Cure Violence' initiative', *Critical Public Health*, 29(2): 146–55.

Roach, J. and Pease, K. (2013) *Evolution and Crime*, Oxford: Routledge.

Roberts, M., Buckland, G. and Redgrave, H. (2019) 'Examining the youth justice system: what drove the falls in first time entrants and custody, and what should we do as a result?', Available from: https://static.wixstatic.com/ugd/b9cf6c_69afbe2836954 4c7bca350229d0be59f.pdf [Accessed 22 November 2024].

Room, R. (2005) 'Stigma, social inequality and alcohol and drug use', *Drug and Alcohol Review*, 24(2): 143–55.

Rose, R. (1971) 'The making of cabinet ministers', *British Journal of Political Science*, 1(4): 393–414.

Royal Commission on the Constitution (Kilbrandon Commission) (1973) *Report of the Royal Commission on the Constitution* (Kilbrandon Report), London: HMSO.

Sampson, R.J. and Laub, J.H. (1993) *Crime in the Making: Pathways and turning points through life*, Cambridge, MA: Harvard University Press.

Sayer, A. (2005) *The Moral Significance of Class*, Cambridge: Cambridge University Press.

Scottish Executive (2000) *It's a Criminal Waste: Stop youth crime now: Report of the Advisory Group on Youth Crime*, Edinburgh: Scottish Executive.

Scottish Executive (2006) *Getting It Right For Every Child: Implementation plan*, Edinburgh: Scottish Executive.

Scottish Government (2008a) *Achieving our Potential: A framework to tackle poverty and income inequality in Scotland*, Edinburgh: Scottish Government.

Scottish Government (2008b) *Equally Well: Report of Ministerial Task Force on Health Inequalities*, Edinburgh: Scottish Government.

Scottish Government (2008c) *Preventing Offending by Young People: A framework for action*, Edinburgh: Scottish Government.

Scottish Government (2019) *Non-sexual Violence in Scotland: Crime and justice*, Edinburgh: Scottish Government.

Scottish Violence Reduction Unit (2020) *Violence is Preventable, not Inevitable: The story and impact of the Scottish Violence Reduction Unit*, Glasgow: SVRU, Available from: http://www.svru.co.uk/wp-content/uploads/2020/02/VRU_Report_Digital_Extra_Lightweight.pdf [Accessed 22 November 2024].

Seenan, G. (2005) 'Scotland has second highest murder rate in Europe', *The Guardian*, 26 September 2005, Available from: https://www.theguardian.com/uk/2005/sep/26/ukcrime.scotland [Accessed 22 November 2024].

Shepherd, J., Avery, V. and Rahman, S. (2016) 'Targeted Policing', *Police Professional*, 28 April, Available from: https://www.cardiff.ac.uk/__data/assets/pdf_file/0006/300669/PP-JPS-2016-article-Targeted-Policing.pdf [Accessed 27 January 2025].

Sloper, P. (2004) 'Facilitators and barriers for co-ordinated multi-agency services', *Childcare, Health and Development*, 30(6): 571–80.

Smith, D. (2000) 'Learning from the Scottish juvenile justice system', *Probation Journal*, 47(1): 12–17.

Smith, D. and Grierson, J. (2018) 'Donald Trump says London hospital is like "war zone" because of knife crime', *The Guardian*, 4 May 2018, Available from: https://www.theguardian.com/us-news/2018/may/04/trump-nra-london-hospital-knives [Accessed 22 November 2024].

Solomon, M. (2019) 'Becoming comfortable with chaos: making collaborative multi-agency working work', *Emotional and Behavioural Difficulties*, 24(4): 391–404.

Spicer, J., Leah, M. and Coomber, R. (2020) 'The variable and evolving nature of "cuckooing" as a form of criminal exploitation in street level drug markets', *Trends in Organised Crime*, 23(4): 301–23.

Standring, A. (2017) 'Evidence-based policymaking and the politics of neoliberal reason: a response to Newman', *Critical Policy Studies*, 11(2): 227–34.

Stehlik, T., Carter, J., Price, D. and Comber, B. (2020) 'Hanging out in the city of tomorrow: a participatory approach to researching the importance of music and arts in the lifeworlds of young people', *Pastoral Care in Education*, 38(3): 273–89.

Stephenson, W. (1935) 'Technique of factor analysis', *Nature*, 136: 297.

Stern, J. (2003) *Terror in the Name of God: Why religious militants kill*, New York, NY: HarperCollins.

Stevens, A., Billingham, L., Schreeche-Powell, E. and Irwin-Rogers, K. (2025) Interventionitis in the criminal justice system: three English case reports, *Critical Criminology*, Available from: https://doi.org/10.1007/s10612-024-09808-x [Accessed 21 March 2025].

Stevenson, M. (2023) 'Cause, effect and the structure of the social world', *Boston University Law Review*, 103: 2001–47.

Sturgeon, J. and Leygue-Eurieult, E. (2020) '"Needs not deeds": the Scottish Children's Hearing and the enduring legacy of Lord Kilbrandon', *Criminocorpus*, Available from: https://journals.openedition.org/criminocorpus/7257 [Accessed 22 November 2024].

Taylor, C. (2016) *Review of the Youth Justice System in England and Wales*, Cm 9298, London: The Stationery Office.

Thorpe, D., Smith, D., Green, C. and Paley, G. (1980) *Out of Care*, London: Allen & Unwin.

Toropova, A., Myrberg, E. and Johansson, S. (2021) 'Teacher job satisfaction: the importance of school working conditions and teacher characteristics', *Education Review*, 73(1): 71–97.

Tutt, N. (1981) 'A decade of policy', *British Journal of Criminology*, 21(3): 246–56.

Tweedie, K. (2005) 'Scotland tops list of world's most violent countries', *The Times*, 19 September 2005, Available from: https://www.thetimes.com/article/scotland-tops-list-of-worlds-most-violent-countries-b0llsm9cv80 [Accessed 22 November 2024].

Tyler, I. (2020) *Stigma: The Machinery of Inequality*, London: Bloomsbury Publishing.

UK Government (2022) 'PCSC act explanatory notes', Available from: https://www.legislation.gov.uk/ukpga/2022/32/pdfs/ukpgaen_20220032_en.pdf [Accessed 22 November 2024].

UK Parliament (2018) 'Knives: crime', Available from: https://questions-statements.parliament.uk/written-questions/detail/2018-07-23/HL9766 [Accessed 22 November 2024].

US Department of Health and Human Services (1986) 'Surgeon General's Workshop on Violence and Public Health', Available from: https://www.nlm.nih.gov/exhibition/confrontingviolence/materials/OB10998.pdf [Accessed 22 November 2024].

Walsh, C., Razey, K., Sheehan, K., Farrington, C., Hazelden, C., Scott, D., Anderson, P. and Caldwell, F. (2023) *Characteristics of Public Health Approaches for Youth Violence Prevention (PH-VP): A rapid review*, Belfast: Queen's University Belfast.

Watts, S. and Stenner, P. (2012) *Doing Q Methodological Research: Theory, method and interpretation*, London: Sage.

Weale, S. (2020) 'Youth services suffer 70% funding cut in less than a decade', *The Guardian*, 20 January, Available from: www.theguardian.com/soci ety/2020/jan/20/youth-services-suffer-70-funding-cut-in-less-than-a-decade [Accessed 27 January 2025].

Welchman, L. and Hossain, S. (2005) *'Honour': Crimes, paradigms, and violence against women*, London: Bloomsbury Publishing.

White, R. (2013) *Youth Gangs, Violence and Social Respect*, London: Palgrave Macmillan.

Widom, C.S. (1989) 'The cycle of violence', *Science*, 244(4901): 160–6.

Williams, D.J., Currie, D., Linden, W. and Donnelly, P.D. (2014) 'Addressing gang-related violence in Glasgow: a preliminary pragmatic quasi-experimental evaluation of the Community Initiative to Reduce Violence (CIRV)', *Aggression and Violent Behaviour*, 19(6): 686–91.

Williams, P. and Clarke, B. (2018) 'The Black criminal Other as an object of social control', *Social Sciences*, 7(11): 234–52.

Wilkinson, R. and Pickett, K. (2009) *The Spirit Level: Why More Equal Societies Almost Always Do Better*, London: Penguin.

Wilson, D.B., Abt, T., Kimbrell, C. and Johnson, W. (2024) 'Protocol: reducing community violence: a systematic meta-review of what works', *Campbell Systematic Review*, 20(2): e1409.

Winlow, S. and Hall, S. (2013) *Rethinking Social Exclusion: The end of the social?*, London: Sage.

Winlow, S. and Hall, S. (2022) *The Death of the Left: Why we must begin from the beginning again*, Bristol: Bristol University Press.

World Health Organization (no date) 'The VPA approach', Available from: https://www.who.int/groups/violence-prevention-alliance/approach [Accessed 22 November 2024].

Wright, R. and Hughes, L. (2018) 'Sajid Javid to announce public health approach to violent crime', *Financial Times*, 1 October 2018, Available from: https://www.ft.com/content/31ab5ab8-c583-11e8-8670-c5353379f7c2 [Accessed 22 November 2024].

Young, J. (2007) *The Vertigo of Late Modernity*, London: Sage.

Younge, G. (2018) 'The radical lessons of a year reporting on knife crime', *The Guardian*, 21 June 2018, Available from: https://www.theguardian.com/membership/2018/jun/21/radical-lessons-knife-crime-beyond-the-blade [Accessed 22 November 2024].

Youth Endowment Fund (2019) 'Announcing our first grantees and new programmes', Available from: https://youthendowmentfund.org.uk/news/grantees-and-programmes/ [Accessed 22 November 2024].

Youth Endowment Fund (2020) 'What works: preventing children and young people from becoming involved in violence', Available from: https://youthendowmentfund.org.uk/wp-content/uploads/2020/10/YEF_What_Works_Report_FINAL.pdf [Accessed 22 November 2024].

Youth Endowment Fund (2022) 'Systems evidence and gap map', Available from: https://youthendowmentfund.org.uk/wp-content/uploads/2022/06/Systems-EGM-Summary-report-June-2022.pdf [Accessed 22 November 2024].

Youth Endowment Fund (2023) 'Arrested children: How to keep children safe and reduce reoffending', Available from: https://youthendowmentfund.org.uk/wp-content/uploads/2023/12/Arrested-children-How-to-keep-children-safe-and-reduce-reoffending.pdf [Accessed 27 January 2025].

Youth Endowment Fund (2024a) 'Children, violence and vulnerability 2024', Available from: https://youthendowmentfund.org.uk/wp-content/uploads/2024/11/CVV24_R1_OverallViolence.pdf [Accessed 22 November 2024].

Youth Endowment Fund (2024b) 'The Youth Endowment Fund: research lead – underlying causes of violence', Available from: https://youthendowmentfund.org.uk/wp-content/uploads/2024/03/Causes-and-contexts-lead-JD-2024.pdf [Accessed 22 November 2024].

Youth Violence Commission (2018) 'Youth Violence Commission interim report', Available from: https://www.yvcommission.com/_files/ugd/ad2256_d4b4f677734a4a4b86cb5833cfcee53f.pdf [Accessed 22 November 2024].

Index

A

accountability 117, 135
Achieving Our Potential framework 36
adverse childhood experiences (ACEs) 9, 51, 66, 107
Advisory Group on Youth Crime (Scotland) 30
antisocial behaviour 30, 38, 43
Atkins, Victoria 52–53
'at-risk' individuals 15, 33, 35, 38, 59, 111, 143
austerity 38–39, 66, 81, 87, 108, 114, 141

B

Bellis, M. 4, 9, 67–68
Billingham, L. 3, 16, 69, 129
biological factors in violence causation 9–10
Braverman, Suella 68–69, 70
Brierley, A. 138
Burnham, Andy 125
Butler, Dawn 70

C

Cardiff Model 41
Carnochan, John 33, 92
causes of violence 7–15, 34, 38, 56, 84, 142
 see also Four Is framework; primary prevention; root (distal/developmental) causes of violence
Ceasefire initiative (Boston) 34, 35
chief officers of police 62, 68–69, 112
Child First agenda 43
child poverty 65, 134
childhood factors in later violence 9, 51, 66, 107
Children and Young Persons Act 1969 37

'children first, offenders second' 40–41
Children in Custody report 136
Children's Commissioner 136
Children's Hearings System 29–30, 31, 40
Citizens' Advisory Panels 101
City Hall summit on serious violence 47
co-design 101
coding frameworks 19
Cohen, David 50
Coles, E. 31
collaboration 62, 94, 98–99, 141
College of Policing 62
Collins, R. 10
commissioning interventions 67, 82, 85, 105–123
community engagement 35, 99–102
community safety partnerships 48, 79, 82, 112
community-level drivers of violence 10–12, 15, 146
Conservative Party 37, 38, 43
Conservative–Liberal Democrat coalition government 39
co-ordination 31, 56, 57
 see also multi-agency working
county lines 48, 99
Crime and Disorder Act 1998 38
cultural changes 35
Cure Violence (CV) 35
Currie, E. 145

D

data coding (research) 19
data gathering for evaluation 56, 59, 80, 110–111, 117, 118–120
data quality concerns 98, 121
data sharing 97–99, 127
Davey, Sir Ed 53
deterrence 34–35
developmental criminology 9

Index

Dick, Cressida 47
direct causes of violence 10
diversion 32, 39–40, 113
documentary analysis 19
domestic violence/intimate partner violence 8, 9, 107, 128, 152
Drakeford, Mark 41

E

early intervention 29, 32, 53, 56, 60, 84, 106–114
Early Intervention Foundation 61, 62
Early Intervention Youth Fund 48
Early Years Framework 32
ecological framework 10–15, 64, 143
Economic and Social Research Council (ESRC) 2, 17
economic costs of violence to society 115
economic geography 21
Edinburgh Study of Youth Transitions and Crime 32
education 48, 82, 83, 127, 129
Ellis, A. 12
employment 9, 12, 29, 145
enforcement 56, 63, 68
England and Wales
 adoption of public health approach 27
 documentary analysis 19
 history of public health approach 37–42
 police-recorded crime data 20
 recent developments 44–71
 research in 18
 trends in violence 5–6
 see also Serious Violence Duty; VRUs (Violence Reduction Units)
Equally Well 36
ethics 20–21, 98, 100, 118, 123
evaluations
 benefits of good 122–123
 data gathering for evaluation 56, 59, 80, 110–111, 117, 118–120
 data quality concerns 98, 121
 funding 116–123
 Home Office 79, 107–111, 116–123, 150
 improving evaluation criteria 147–149
 of policy influence 126–127

safeguarding concerns 119–120, 123
statistical significance 36, 41, 148
'toolkits' 61, 62, 109–110, 121, 140
Violence Prevention Alliance 34
VRUs (Violence Reduction Units) 107–108, 116–123, 139, 156–161
Youth Endowment Fund 60–62, 90, 109–110, 121, 140
evidence-based commissioning 63
evidence-based decision making 117
evidence-based interventions 48, 54–55, 58–60, 80, 109–110, 115, 116–123, 140
exclusions from school 99, 127, 129, 135
exploitation 13, 99

F

fear of violence 3, 6
 see also perceptions of community safety
Flyvbjerg, B. 21–22
focus group methods 17–19
Four Is framework
 applying 138–141
 coordinated action 134–138
 holistic public health approach 141–151
 outline of 16–17
 public health approach 45, 64, 67–68
four-step model (WHO) 15, 34, 60, 62, 64, 142
Foxcroft, Vicky 51
Fraser, A. 11, 36, 87, 92, 104, 106
funding
 Early Intervention Youth Fund 48
 evaluations 116–123
 high impact interventions 109–110
 interventions and programmes 136–137
 local policing bodies 62
 London VRU 128–129
 long-term funding 151
 pressure to spend money in haste 79–80, 115–116
 resource pooling 84
 scaling up interventions 115
 Serious Violence Duty 95
 single-year funding 87, 90–91, 151
 and staff retention 87
 Surge (Grip) funding 58, 70

VRUs (Violence Reduction
   Units) 67, 75–80, 82, 87,
   90–91, 106, 111, 115–116
   see also Youth Endowment Fund

G

gangs
   and the 2011 riots 39, 43, 46
   Cure Violence (CV) 35
   and 'mattering' 13
   new court orders 69
   positive alternatives to 57
   support for leaving 35
   zero tolerance initiatives 34
gender 3
generalisability 4
geographic scope 4
Getting it Right for Every Child
   (GIRFEC) (Scottish Executive,
   2006) 31–32
Gilligan, J. 10, 13, 106
Gillon, F. 36, 92, 104, 106, 129
Glasgow 18, 20, 33, 36, 53, 56
grassroots organisations 114, 118
Gray, P. 9
Grip (Surge) funding 58, 70

H

health partners 48
Hewitt, Martin 106
high-impact interventions 59, 62,
   109–110, 121, 140
high-risk individuals 29, 35, 38, 106
holistic approaches 15, 17, 31, 53,
   84, 141–151
Home Affairs Committees 65
Home Office
   definition of public health
      approach 85
   evaluations of VRUs 79, 107–111,
      116–123, 150
   guidance 66
   and the Serious Violence Duty 95
homicides 6, 32, 34, 42, 46–47, 107
Hope Collective 100, 128
hospital data 41, 46–47, 75, 76, 107,
   147, 148
housing 3, 8–9, 13, 127, 138, 145

I

impact measurement 107, 116–123,
   147–148
indicated interventions 106

inequality
   Achieving Our Potential
      framework 36
   causes of violence 8, 10–11, 13,
      65, 66, 107
   domestic violence/intimate partner
      violence 152
   Four Is framework 16, 134–135,
      153–154
   lack of government focus
      on 45, 144
   Scottish VRU 124
information sharing 58, 85, 91,
   97–99, 117
inspections 91
institutions 16, 45, 124–129,
   135–136, 144, 152, 154
interactions/relationships 16, 45, 89,
   92, 137–138, 152, 154
interdepartmental (government)
   cooperation 88
interventions
   domestic violence 152
   Four Is framework 16,
      136–137, 154
   government focus on 45, 66, 137,
      140, 142
   'interventionitis' 137, 140
   scaling up 114–116
   VRUs as commissioners of
      105–123, 125–126
   see also evidence-based
      interventions
interview methods 17–19
Irwin-Rogers, K. 3, 11, 69, 87,
   100, 129

J

Javid, Sajid 52, 54, 59, 61, 70, 83,
   99–100, 125
Johnson, Boris 57, 58
joined-up working 99, 146–147
   see also multi-agency working
Joseph Rowntree Foundation 65

K

key performance indicators
   (KPIs) 117, 139
Khan, Sadiq 27, 47, 49, 52, 55,
   75, 125
Kilbrandon Report (1964) 29–30, 31
knife crime 7, 41–42, 46–47, 49,
   69, 107, 160

Index

Knife Crime Prevention Orders (KCPOs) 69
Krug, E.G. 15, 33, 64, 105, 111

L

Labour Party 1, 37
leadership 91–94
Lloyd, J. 149
local authorities 62, 94
local needs assessments 65, 79, 121, 129
localised programmatic interventions 45, 56, 58
local-level data 41
London
  adoption of public health approach 27, 52
  Glasgow as model for 53, 56
  Inclusion Charter 129
  knife crime 47, 49
  media agendas 42
  police-recorded crime data 8, 20
  reason for focus on 2
  research in 18
  trends in violence 6
  VRUs (Violence Reduction Units) 55–56, 128–129, 147, 150
Longford Report 37
long-term nature of work 57, 82, 105, 108, 112, 139, 149, 151
long-term research 121

M

macro level violence prevention 16, 67–68, 100, 134
Manzoni, J. 98
mattering 12–14, 135, 155
May, Theresa 27, 53–54, 59, 63
McAra, L. 30, 31, 32, 92
McCluskey, Karyn 33, 36, 92
McVie, S. 31, 32, 92
media agendas 42, 46, 48–50
Metropolitan Police Service 6, 8, 20, 47, 56
micro-sociology 10
models of public health implementation 15, 64, 65, 66, 142
multi-agency working
  challenges to 86–88
  competitiveness as barrier to 86–87

continuum of 85
focus in England and Wales on 45, 48, 65, 66, 67, 70
key ingredients to enhance 88–91
leadership 91–94
local coordination 146
moving beyond 149–151
multi-layer governance 88
need for senior-level support 88, 91
safeguarding concerns 149
Serious Violence Duty 61, 62
Serious Violence Strategy 53, 54
versus silo working 84, 140
VRUs (Violence Reduction Units) 55–56, 58, 59, 79, 83–94, 146–147

N

New Labour 19, 30, 38–40
New Public Management (NPM) 116, 150
NHS England 49

O

Office for National Statistics 5, 6, 7, 136
Organisation for Economic Co-operation and Development (OECD) 65, 134
outcomes 48, 84, 87, 107–108, 117, 136, 143, 147
Owens, R. 149

P

partnership working
  building legitimacy and securing trust 81–83
  leadership 91–94
  Serious Violence Duty 62
  Serious Violence Strategy 47, 48
  VRUs (Violence Reduction Units) 56, 60, 79, 85, 124
  see also multi-agency working
Patel, Priti 57, 58, 68
Pease, K. 10
perceptions of community safety 6, 35–36, 148–149, 160
Philp, Chris 84
Pinker, S. 5
Police, Crime, Sentencing and Courts Act 2022 61–63, 94, 96, 97, 99

police and crime commissioners 48, 57, 75, 112
Police Scotland 54
police-recorded crime data 20, 41, 42, 70
policing 34, 39, 49, 50, 58, 68–69, 109
policy change 67, 85, 123–129, 141–145, 151
poverty as cause of violence 3, 8, 10–11, 13, 36, 57, 65, 107, 128, 149
Preventing Offending by Young People (Scottish Government 2008) 32
primary prevention 15, 105, 106–114, 139, 143, 147, 149
problem-oriented policing 34, 58
professional networks 83, 89
programmatic interventions 45, 63, 65, 67, 137, 142, 143–144, 146
protective factors 9
psychological tension 12, 13–14
public health approach
  competing conceptions of 45, 51–52
  consensus 52–53
  geographic scope 4
  history in England and Wales 37–42
  history in Scotland 27–36
  holistic approaches 15, 17, 31, 53, 84, 141–151
  institutionalisation in London 55–63
  limitations of existing interpretations 14–15
  media calls for 49
  mismatch between rhetoric and actuality 66
  'new public health duty' 61
  overview 14–17
  recent developments in England and Wales 44–71
  research 17–21
  Serious Violence Strategy (Home Office 2018) 47–48
  shifting language away from 70–71
  violence affecting young people 3
Public Health England 66
Public Health, Youth and Violence Reduction (PHYVR) project 16, 17–21, 93, 134, 156–161

public opinions on crime 6–7, 113
  see also perceptions of community safety
'punitive prevention' 45, 68
punitive responses 30, 31, 37, 39, 45, 68–70

Q
Q-grid activity 156–161

R
racial discrimination 29, 39, 124, 135
Rae, Sir Willie 33
randomised controlled trials 60, 109, 119, 121
referral orders 40
relational poverty 138
relationships as micro-level prevention 16, 91–92
  see also interactions/relationships
reoffending 54
research ethics 20–21
resource pooling 84
restorative justice 40
riots (2011) 39, 43, 46
'risk factors' 9, 38, 66
Roach, J. 10
root (distal/developmental) causes of violence 8–10, 53, 66, 114, 124, 127, 145
Rudd, Amber 47

S
safeguarding concerns 119–120, 123, 149
schools 82–83, 99, 127, 129, 135–136, 145
Scotland
  crime rates 32
  decline in violence 2006–2015 17, 27, 36
  documentary analysis 19
  early roots of public health approach 29–36
  Getting it Right for Every Child (GIRFEC) 31–32
  police-recorded crime data 20
  policy influence of VRU 124
  prevention 106
  public health approach as model for England 49–50, 51, 53, 58, 125
  research in 18

Index

stable rates since 2014 41
systems guidance 92
VRUs (Violence Reduction Units) 92, 124, 150
Scottish National Party (SNP) 31–32
secondary prevention 15, 105, 109, 113, 143
Serious Violence Duty 55–63, 65, 67, 70, 94–99, 127–128, 140–141, 147
Serious Violence Reduction Orders (SVROs) 69
Serious Violence Strategy (Home Office 2018) 47–48, 51, 52, 54, 61
shame and humiliation 12–14, 135, 152, 155
Shepherd, J. 41
short-termism 105, 109, 111, 137, 139, 147, 160
see also single-year funding
single-year funding 87, 90–91, 151
social and economic injustices 61
social infrastructure 135–136
Social Investment Business 61
Social Work (Scotland) Act 1968 29–30
societal-level causes of violence 10–12, 15, 65, 146
staff recruitment 58, 78, 83, 90
staff retention 87, 90
staff training 31, 90
stages of prevention 15, 64, 142
stakeholder engagement 99–102, 112, 117, 141
statistical significance 33, 36, 41, 148
statistics on crime 4, 5–8, 36, 41–42, 46–48
see also hospital data; police-recorded crime data
Stephenson, W. 156
Stevens, A. 137
Stevenson, M. 146
stigma 9, 135
stop-and-search 39, 50, 68–69, 70, 135
strategic needs assessments 65, 79, 121, 129
Strathclyde Police Force 33, 36, 54
stress regulation 9
structural change 137

structural drivers of violence 3, 12, 16, 56, 66, 100, 124
structural humiliation 12, 135
substance abuse 10–11
Surge (Grip) funding 58, 70
systems guidance 61, 140
systems leadership 91–92, 93, 94

T

tailored approaches 85
Taylor, Charlie 40
tertiary prevention 15, 105, 108, 109, 113, 120–121, 143
theories of change 122
third sector organisations 61, 81, 114, 137
timeliness of evidence 121
'toolkits' 61, 62, 109–110, 121, 140
'tough' approaches 30, 38–40, 43, 63, 68, 70
trauma 9, 50, 51, 90, 92
trends in violence 5–8
Trump, Donald 48–49

U

United Nations Convention on the Rights of the Child 31
universal interventions 106, 111
University of Glasgow 20–21
US 4, 14–15, 17, 28–29, 33–36, 48, 60, 141

V

Violence Prevention Alliance 34
VRUs (Violence Reduction Units)
building legitimacy and securing trust 81–83
centralised versus hub and spoke structures 76–79
commissioning interventions 67, 82, 85, 105–123
director backgrounds 77–78
England and Wales 55–63
establishing 76–79
form and focus of 55–59
Four Is framework 139
future of 146–151
Home Office evaluations of 79, 107–111, 116–123, 150
hybrid structures 78–79
local needs assessments 65, 79, 121, 129

London 52, 54, 55, 75
mandatory requirements 79
pressure to spend money in haste 79–81, 115
research interviews 18
response strategies 79
Scotland 32–33, 51, 106
and the Serious Violence Duty 95–97
statistics on effectiveness 35
workshops (research method) 20
Youth Violence Commission 67

W

Wales 40–41
Walsh, C. 15
weapon carrying 36, 41–42, 69
'what works' paradigms 38, 55–56, 109, 121, 137
'when' prevention happens 15
WHO (World Health Organization) 10–12, 13, 15, 32, 33–36, 58, 60, 62, 64, 65, 80, 105, 111, 142, 145
whole child approaches 31, 58
whole-system approach 32, 66, 70, 85, 92, 93
'working with' approaches 102
workshops (research method) 20, 156–161
World Report on Violence and Health (WHO 2002) 33–34

Y

Young Londoners Fund 57
young people, engaging with 99–102
Younge, Gary 49
youth (juvenile) justice systems 29–30, 37–38, 40–41, 145
youth custodial institutions 37, 39, 136
Youth Endowment Fund 3, 7, 54, 59–61, 67, 109–110, 121, 137, 139–140
Youth Justice Board 40, 49, 126
Youth Justice Criminal Evidence Act 1999 38
youth services/youth work 66, 135, 138, 145
Youth Violence Commission 50–52, 67, 92